Is Athlete Drug Testing Needed?

Lydia Bjornlund

INCONTROVERSY

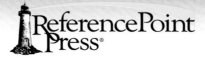
ReferencePoint
Press®

San Diego, CA

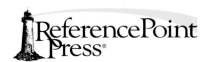

© 2014 ReferencePoint Press, Inc.
Printed in the United States

For more information, contact:
ReferencePoint Press, Inc.
PO Box 27779
San Diego, CA 92198
www. ReferencePointPress.com

LIBRARY OF CONGRESS CATALOGING-IN-PUBLICATION DATA

Bjornlund, Lydia, 1961–
  Is athlete drug testing needed? / by Lydia Bjornlund.
    pages cm. -- (In controversy)
  Audience: Grade 9 to 12.
  Includes bibliographical references and index.
  ISBN-13: 978-1-60152-554-3 (hardback)
  ISBN-10: 1-60152-554-0 (hardback)
 1. Drug testing--Popular works. 2. Doping in sports--Popular works. I. Title.
  HV5823.B56   2014
  362.29'164--dc23
                                                          2013011824

Contents

Foreword

I n 2008, as the US economy and economies worldwide were falling into the worst recession since the Great Depression, most Americans had difficulty comprehending the complexity, magnitude, and scope of what was happening. As is often the case with a complex, controversial issue such as this historic global economic recession, looking at the problem as a whole can be overwhelming and often does not lead to understanding. One way to better comprehend such a large issue or event is to break it into smaller parts. The intricacies of global economic recession may be difficult to understand, but one can gain insight by instead beginning with an individual contributing factor, such as the real estate market. When examined through a narrower lens, complex issues become clearer and easier to evaluate.

This is the idea behind ReferencePoint Press's *In Controversy* series. The series examines the complex, controversial issues of the day by breaking them into smaller pieces. Rather than looking at the stem cell research debate as a whole, a title would examine an important aspect of the debate such as *Is Stem Cell Research Necessary?* or *Is Embryonic Stem Cell Research Ethical?* By studying the central issues of the debate individually, researchers gain a more solid and focused understanding of the topic as a whole.

Each book in the series provides a clear, insightful discussion of the issues, integrating facts and a variety of contrasting opinions for a solid, balanced perspective. Personal accounts and direct quotes from academic and professional experts, advocacy groups, politicians, and others enhance the narrative. Sidebars add depth to the discussion by expanding on important ideas and events. For quick reference, a list of key facts concludes every chapter. Source notes, an annotated organizations list, bibliography, and index provide student researchers with additional tools for papers and class discussion.

The *In Controversy* series also challenges students to think critically about issues, to improve their problem-solving skills, and to sharpen their ability to form educated opinions. As President Barack Obama stated in a March 2009 speech, success in the twenty-first century will not be measurable merely by students' ability to "fill in a bubble on a test but whether they possess 21st century skills like problem-solving and critical thinking and entrepreneurship and creativity." Those who possess these skills will have a strong foundation for whatever lies ahead.

No one can know for certain what sort of world awaits today's students. What we can assume, however, is that those who are inquisitive about a wide range of issues; open-minded to divergent views; aware of bias and opinion; and able to reason, reflect, and reconsider will be best prepared for the future. As the international development organization Oxfam notes, "Today's young people will grow up to be the citizens of the future: but what that future holds for them is uncertain. We can be quite confident, however, that they will be faced with decisions about a wide range of issues on which people have differing, contradictory views. If they are to develop as global citizens all young people should have the opportunity to engage with these controversial issues."

In Controversy helps today's students better prepare for tomorrow. An understanding of the complex issues that drive our world and the ability to think critically about them are essential components of contributing, competing, and succeeding in the twenty-first century.

A Universal Dilemma

On January 14, 2013, US cyclist Lance Armstrong admitted in a taped interview with former talk-show host Oprah Winfrey that he had used banned performance-enhancing drugs during competition. Armstrong had won the grueling Tour de France race in seven consecutive years from 1999 to 2005. By his own admission, Armstrong had used anabolic steroids, human growth hormone, and erythropoietin (EPO), another hormone. Armstrong attributed his actions to a "ruthless desire to win" and said he did not consider it cheating. "I viewed it as a level playing field,"[1] he told Winfrey.

The confession came as a shock to many because Armstrong had spent more than a decade vehemently refuting allegations of doping. Six months before Armstrong's admission, the United States Anti-Doping Agency (USADA) had issued a one-thousand-page report that accused Armstrong not only of doping but of masterminding "the most sophisticated, professionalized and successful doping programme the sport has ever seen."[2] Armstrong was stripped of his Tour de France titles and banned from further competition. The evidence compiled against him included testimony from several teammates who claimed that if they did not go along with Armstrong's plan, they found themselves without a job. Notably missing from the evidence against Armstrong were positive readings on drug tests.

For two decades Armstrong had repeatedly passed the tests administered to identify substances banned by the International Cycling Union (Union Cycliste Internationale, or UCI), the governing body for sports cycling that oversees international competitions. Teammates say that one reason Armstrong passed is that team doctors were often one step ahead of the tests. "We were able to cheat throughout the whole '99 tour [Tour de France] by probably every third or fourth day taking a shot of EPO,"[3] says Tyler Hamilton, who was on Armstrong's cycling team. EPO, a hormone that is naturally produced by the kidneys and stimulates the production of red blood cells, increases the blood's oxygen-carrying capacity and therefore increases endurance. Many cyclists say this gives them the endurance to stay in the race. In addition to these doping allegations, some people believe that Armstrong had found ways to discern when drug tests were scheduled, even speculating that he made charitable donations to the UCI in exchange for information about its drug-testing protocol.

For critics of athlete drug testing, Armstrong's case points to serious problems with the practice. These critics argue that elite athletes like Armstrong will always find a way around the tests. Advocates of drug testing, on the other hand, say that the case reinforces the need for stringent enforcement of policies regarding the use of performance-enhancing drugs and vigilance about drug testing.

"Winning at all cost is big money. This has made the world of sports so competitive that the inevitable was sure to come along—cheating."[7]

— Robert A. Stinchcomb, athletic director.

New Light on an Old Controversy

Allegations of drug use in the Tour de France are nothing new. "For as long as the Tour has existed, since 1903, its participants have been doping themselves," says Hans Halter, a German journalist and physician. "The Tour, in fact, is only possible because—not despite the fact—there is doping."[4] Cyclists who have been caught using performance-enhancing drugs consistently argue that a rider cannot win without the edge the drugs provide. As part of a plea bargain in In October 2012, George Hincapie, a member of Armstrong's team, confessed to using drugs, putting an end to his eighteen-year career as a professional cyclist. "Early in my professional career, it became clear to me that, given the widespread use of performance-enhancing drugs by cyclists at the top of the profession, it was not possible to compete at the highest level without them,"[5] he explains. Swiss rider Alex Zulle compares doping on the Tour de France like driving on the highway. "The law says there's a speed limit of 65, but everyone is driving 70 or faster. Why should I be the one who obeys the speed limit? So I had two alternatives: either fit in and go along with the others or go back to being a house painter."[6]

Tour de France cyclists rely on performance-enhancing drugs to obtain the stamina they need to endure twenty-one straight days of cycling through the French countryside. For many years amphetamines were the drug of choice. Amphetamines stimulate the brain areas associated with vigilance, mood, and alertness by releasing norepinephrine, a substance stored in nerve endings, which speeds up the heart and the metabolism. Cyclists, runners, and other athletes in search of alertness and speed often rely on amphetamines. Amphetamines were among the first classes of drugs banned by athletic regulatory organizations.

By the late 1980s amphetamines had been replaced by EPO,

Lance Armstrong, celebrating his seventeenth-stage victory in the 2004 Tour de France, outwitted drug tests for years before publicly admitting to using performance-enhancing drugs. The Armstrong case has prompted calls for increased vigilance against doping athletes.

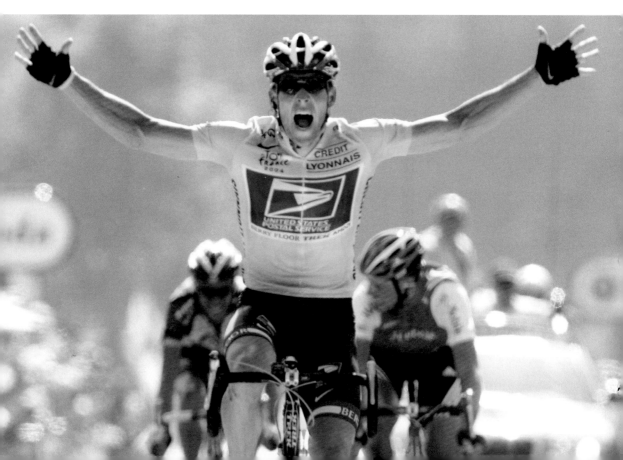

a hormone that is naturally produced by the kidneys and stimulates the production of red blood cells, which increases the blood's oxygen-carrying capacity and therefore increases endurance. Drug testers were slow to respond to this new development; it took a decade before a reliable test for EPO was created, and even then elite athletes found ways to beat the system.

Blood doping is also used by athletes to enhance performance. With blood doping an athlete boosts the number of red blood cells by having healthy blood removed when his or her body is rested and then transfused back into the athlete when needed for competition. The first known case of blood doping occurred at the 1980 Summer Olympics, when Finnish long-distance runner Kaarlo Maaninka was transfused with two pints of blood before two medal-winning races. Blood doping was added to the International Olympic Committee's (IOC) list of banned procedures in 1986 and is prohibited by most athletic organizations.

Another class of drugs targeted by athletic organizations is anabolic (muscle-building) steroids. Like EPO, steroids are found naturally in the human body, but anabolic steroids, which were first produced in 1953, have three to five times the muscle-building effects of natural testosterone. Steroids stimulate the body to grow muscle; any sport in which muscle and strength are advantages is vulnerable to steroid abuse. Steroids were widely used at the Olympic Games in the 1950s and were first banned by the IOC in 1975. In 1981 the use of steroids became illegal without a doctor's prescription. Steroids can be difficult to detect, however, because there are literally hundreds of different types, many of which are so-called designer drugs, a term that refers to drugs that have been created illegally for distribution on the black market.

The most recent challenge for drug testers is human growth hormone (HGH). HGH was first used in the 1950s as a treatment for children who failed to grow due to a growth hormone deficiency. HGH gives a sudden burst of energy and has been shown to improve sprinting ability, particularly when combined

"The downfall of Olympic heroes has cast a cloud of suspicion over sports. And the dopers' victims aren't just the rivals from whom they stole their golden podium moments but every clean athlete whose performance is greeted with skepticism."[8]

— Christie Aschwanden, sports journalist.

with anabolic steroids. Human growth hormone has been banned by most athletic organizations, but because it occurs naturally in the human body, it is difficult to detect. Athletic organizations believe athletes have been using HGH, often in combination with steroids, for decades, but the first case in which a drug test led to an athlete being sanctioned occurred in 2009.

Drug tests today are designed to detect all of these classes of drugs, but even in the most regulated sports, drug use continues among athletes. "Winning at all cost is big money," says Robert A. Stinchcomb, athletic director of the Darlington School in Rome, Georgia, who published an article warning coaches about performance-enhancing drugs. "This has made the world of sports so competitive that the inevitable was sure to come along—cheating."[7]

Given the publicity surrounding drug use among elite athletes, sports fans justifiably have begun to assume that the athletes who win races and smash long-standing records must be taking something to give them that superiority. "The downfall of Olympic heroes has cast a cloud of suspicion over sports," writes Christie Aschwanden in a 2012 article in *Smithsonian* magazine. "And the dopers' victims aren't just the rivals from whom they stole their golden podium moments but every clean athlete whose performance is greeted with skepticism."[8]

Many athletes are frustrated by this skepticism. "I am not some kind of crusader, but I get really angry when I hear that behind every athletic success there is doping," says George Mavrotas, a former Olympic water polo athlete and Hellenic Olympic Committee commissioner. "Even if the revealed doping cases are few, they are enough to spoil the picture of the sport." Mavrotas is among the many athletes who want more frequent, more reliable, and more comprehensive tests to keep drugs from becoming a part of athletics. "Antidoping procedures must be considered by athletes as part of their training and competition routine,"[9] he says.

Clean athletes often believe that drug testing not only ensures a more level playing field, but also is the only way to prove that

"I am not some kind of crusader, but I get really angry when I hear that behind every athletic success there is doping. Even if the revealed doping cases are few, they are enough to spoil the picture of the sport."[9]

— George Mavrotas, Olympic water polo athlete.

they have earned their success without breaking the rules. "I get tested all the time," says Rebecca Adlington, a British swimmer who won two gold medals at the 2008 Olympic Games. "At the Olympics you are tested every time you race and have to have blood tests. I did blood profiling before the Olympics as well so that if anybody ever said 'she's on drugs' I can prove I'm not. I'm not and never will be. I don't . . . believe in it."[10] In today's environment in which athletes continue to deny drug use even as the evidence against them mounts up, submitting to tests frequently and regularly may be the only way to convince a skeptical public that they are honest.

Facts

- In the month following Lance Armstrong's confession to using performance-enhancing drugs, 39 percent of visitors to an ESPN site on the story agreed that Armstrong's lifetime ban should be shortened if he cooperates fully with cycling authorities.

- More than one hundred different types of anabolic steroids have been developed. Most synthetic anabolic steroids have one hundred times as much testosterone as is produced naturally by an adult male.

- Erythropoietin is injected under the skin and can boost red blood cell count for six weeks or longer. It has been shown to increase the oxygen supply by as much as 7 to 10 percent.

CHAPTER ONE

What Are the Origins of the Athlete Drug-Testing Controversy?

Athletes have always looked for new ways to get an edge on the competition. The earliest references to using drugs for this purpose date back almost three thousand years to the first Olympics, when competitors boosted their testosterone levels by eating crushed sheep testicles. Roman gladiators took hallucinogens and stimulants to stave off fatigue. In ancient civilizations of South America, athletes chewed coca leaves—from which cocaine is derived—to make them more alert and alleviate pain.

For most of Olympic history, using drugs was not considered cheating. Elite athletes at the Olympics and other international sporting competitions often used potent mixtures of cocaine, heroin, and strychnine to gain an edge over the competition. Thomas Hicks won the marathon in the 1904 Olympic Games aided by doses of brandy and injections of strychnine—a mixture that nearly killed him.

By the 1920s it had become evident to athletic organizations that restrictions regarding drug use in sport were needed. In 1928 the International Association of Athletics Federation (IAAF), the governing body for international track and field competitions, became the first international sports organization to prohibit doping. Other athletic organizations followed suit, but the bans were largely ineffective because they were not enforced by drug testing.

The twentieth century ushered in new performance-enhancing drugs, most notably anabolic steroids. Olympic athletes saw that the use of performance-enhancing drugs could help immensely in the quest for a medal; professional athletes grew to believe that their very careers depended on taking drugs that would allow them to have the strength, endurance, and/or alertness to excel in their sport. So performance-enhancing drugs increasingly became a part of sports.

Controversy Leads to Drug Testing

With the growing use of drugs came the growing risk to athletes, and several high-profile incidents attracted the attention of athletic organizers. At the 1960 Olympic Games in Rome, Danish cyclist Knud Enemark Jensen collapsed during a race and later died. An autopsy showed that he was under the influence of amphetamines, which had caused him to lose consciousness.

Over the next several years the urgency of the effort to rid sports of dangerous drugs was highlighted by several other widely publicized incidents, including the July 1967 death of British cyclist Tom Simpson during the Tour de France. Simpson, who once said, "If it takes ten to kill you, take nine and win,"[11] had taken amphetamines and brandy during the race to combat the symptoms of a stomach bug. Also in 1967 runner Dick Howard died of a heroin overdose. In 1968 German boxer Jupp Elze died after a cocktail of amphetamines.

The sudden and dramatic deaths of these elite athletes caused the sports world to take notice. For the first time, sports federations for both professional and amateur athletic organizations began to pass more stringent regulations regarding drugs and establish tests to enforce the bans. In 1966 UCI (cycling) and the Fédération Internationale de Football Association (FIFA), which rules international soccer events, became the first international sports orga-

WADA and the Spirit of the Game

In the aftermath of public doping scandals, the First World Conference on Doping in Sport was convened in February 1999. From this meeting came the World Anti-Doping Agency, which was established as an independent international agency to oversee antidoping strategies for the Olympic Games. After extensive consultation with sports authorities worldwide, WADA introduced the first World Anti-Doping Code in 2002. The purposes of the Code and the program it supports are twofold: to protect the right of athletes to participate in competitions that are free of doping, thus protecting both the health of athletes and the fairness of the competition and to ensure coordinated anti-doping programs that include detection, deterrence, and prevention.

WADA defines the spirit of sport as "the celebration of human spirit, body and mind, is characterized by the following values:

- Ethics, fair play and honesty
- Health
- Excellence in performance
- Character and education
- Fun and joy
- Teamwork
- Dedication and commitment
- Respect for rules and laws
- Respect for self and other participants
- Courage
- Community and solidarity."

WADA, "World Anti-Doping Code: 2007 Code Amendments," p. 8. www.wada-ama.org.

nizations to introduce doping tests in their world championship competitions. The IOC followed suit the next year by creating a list of prohibited substances and setting up an independent medical commission to oversee the testing process. The first compulsory drug tests for Olympic athletes took place at the 1968 Winter Games in Grenoble, France, and the Summer Games in Mexico City that same year. During the latter, Sweden's Hans-Gunnar Liljenwall, who competed in the pentathlon, earned the dubious distinction of becoming the first Olympic athlete to test positive for using a banned substance and was stripped of his bronze medal. Liljenwall said he had drunk two beers to calm his nerves during the pistol shooting part of the pentathlon competition.

The first full-scale drug-testing program for Olympic athletes took place four years later at the 1972 Olympic Games. In the Winter Games seven athletes tested positive for banned substances, including American Rick DeMont, who tested positive for the stimulant ephedrine after winning the 400-meter freestyle. Over the next several games the number of athletes testing positive for banned substances increased as new and more rigorous controls were put in place. The IOC added anabolic steroids to the list of banned substances and methods in 1975 and began testing athletes for steroid use at the 1976 Olympic Games in Montreal.

Several other federations for elite athletics joined the IOC in banning performance-enhancing substances and testing for their use. Results varied considerably, however. The testing program undertaken by the UCI, which began in 1966, did not result in a single positive drug test for over three decades—until after a drug bust brought worldwide attention to doping in elite cycling. In this 1998 event, a raid by the French police caught cyclists using substances that were not only banned by the UCI but also against the law in France. In 1963 France had enacted an antidoping law, becoming the first country to do so, but the 1998 raid was the first time athletes had been arrested under the law.

The Tour de France scandal highlighted the need for an independent international agency that would set unified standards for antidoping work and coordinate the efforts of sports organizations and public authorities. The IOC took the initiative and convened the First World Conference on Doping in Sport in Lausanne, Switzerland, in February 1999. Following the recommendation of the conference, the World Anti-Doping Agency (WADA) was established on November 10, 1999.

Early Criticism

As drug-testing programs emerged and the tests themselves evolved, critics argued that they gave rise to a new set of circumstances that were unfair to athletes. In the 1968 Olympics, for instance, only one athlete tested positive for a banned substance, but fourteen other athletes tested positive for tranquilizers that were not yet on the IOC's list of prohibited substances. Critics argue that the list of banned substances is always behind the curve, resulting in inequities because testing organizations may disqualify an athlete who is using a banned substance, while athletes using substances that have a greater influence on performance are allowed to continue because there is no way to test for those substances. Whether there

East German swimmers rejoice after winning a gold medal in 1976 in the women's 4x100-meter relay. Classified documents released years later revealed that many of East Germany's women swimmers were using steroids.

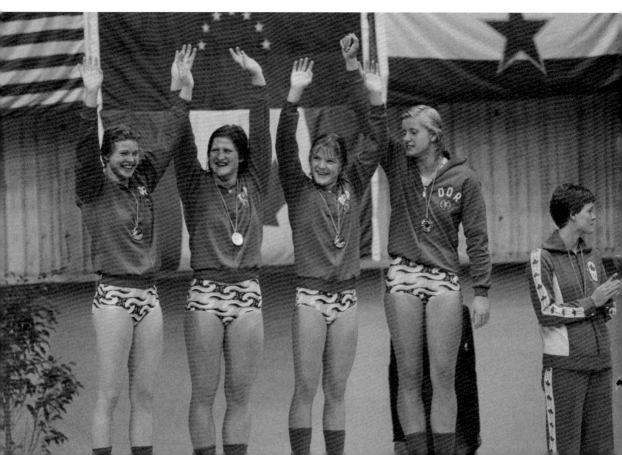

should be retroactive punishments for these drugs remains at issue. It took decades to develop a reliable test for anabolic steroids, which were widely used by athletes in strength competitions. In 1974 a test was created, and steroids were added to the IOC's list of banned substances. According to WADA, the tests "resulted in a marked increase in the number of doping-related disqualifications in the late 1970s, notably in strength-related sports such as throwing events and weightlifting."[12]

Even with the tests, however, drug use was often difficult to prove. At the 1976 Olympics, East German women swimmers won eleven of the thirteen individual gold medals and set eight world records in the process, but none of the swimmers tested positive for steroids. American swimmer Shirley Babashoff, a gold medal hopeful, complained at the time of cheating among the East Germans. "They had gotten so big, and when we heard their voices, we thought we were in a coed locker room," she recalled in 2004. "I don't know why it wasn't obvious to other people, too."[13]

Classified documents released after the fall of the Berlin Wall thirteen years later confirmed Babashoff's claims, but the tests at the time of the competition were inadequate to detect the type of steroids used by the East German team. As the drug tests became more comprehensive, drug makers continued to develop new drugs that would not be detected. The IOC simply could not keep pace. "Through the 1980s and 1990s, clandestine doping programs spread from sport to sport guided by modern, albeit unethical, pharmacists and sports medicine professionals," write researchers David A. Baron, David M. Martin, and Samir Abol Magd in a 2007 article reviewing the increase of performance-enhancing drug use worldwide. "Doping became so prevalent in Olympic sport that some argued that all records should be discarded or put on hold until all forms of doping could be detected and stopped."[14]

Perhaps the most memorable case of cheating at the Olympic Games was that of Canadian sprinter Ben Johnson. Johnson won the 100-meter sprint at the 1988 Olympic Games in Seoul, South Korea, shattering the world record by a full one-tenth of a second. But his drug test found stanozolol, an anabolic steroid, in his urine. Johnson was stripped of his medal and suspended from the sport. He attempted a comeback in 1991 but again tested positive for banned substances in 1993 and was permanently banned from competition.

The gold medal at the 1988 Olympics went to second-place finisher Carl Lewis, who had himself tested positive for banned substances prior to the Olympics. The high-profile incident shed light on the extent of drug use among Olympic athletes and caused many people to begin to question the efficacy and fairness of the IOC's drug policies. Subsequent events revealed that six of the eight runners in the final 100-meter sprint at the 1988 Olympic Games had used banned substances at one time or another.

New Doping Methods Require New Tests

Critics of outlawing performance-enhancing drugs in sports say that it is impossible for the tests to keep up with the drugs, particularly given the variances that are possible with steroids. As soon as a test is developed for one drug, another takes its place. In 2002 scientists began experimenting with a new group of synthetic steroids designed to be undetectable by drug tests. These so-called

Canadian sprinter Ben Johnson breaks from the pack for a record-setting win of the 100-meter race at the 1988 Olympics. Johnson was stripped of his medal after testing positive for steroids. He was eventually banned from all competition after later tests confirmed ongoing use of banned substances.

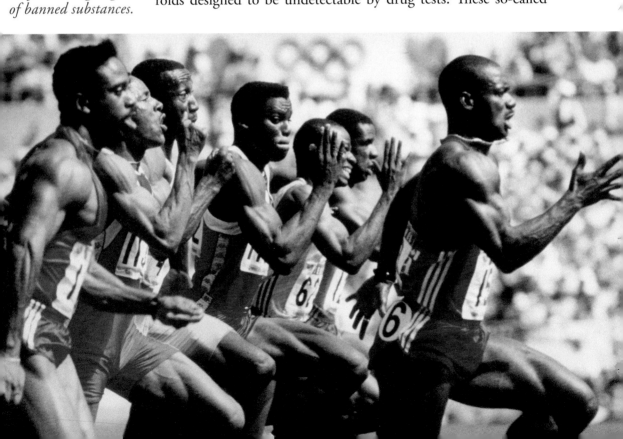

designer steroids are intended for use by athletes and have no approved medical use. The drugs include desoxymethyltestosterone (Madol), norbolethone (Genabol), and tetrahydrogestrinone (THG), a steroid that athletes nicknamed "the clear" because it could not be detected by drug tests.

A test has been developed for "the clear," but experts say that a new threat is on the horizon: fast-acting steroids. These synthetic testosterones are not as powerful as anabolic steroids, but they can help speed recovery and enhance workouts. They also clear the body faster, which makes them harder to detect in drug testing.

Another challenge for the makers of drug tests is that many of the substances used to enhance performance are found naturally in the body in small quantities, which makes them hard to detect. Human growth hormone (HGH), which athletes began to take in the 1990s to boost their performance, is one example. David Howman, director general of WADA, called HGH "one of the biggest threats to sport right now and has been for many years. Athletes have taken it with impunity because it was not detectable."[15]

Tests for HGH have been developed recently, however, and yielded the first positive result in 2009, when a test detected unusually high levels of HGH in the urine of British rugby player Terry Newton. The next year, Mike Jacobs, a first baseman in the Colorado Rockies organization, became the first professional athlete in the United States to test positive for HGH. After being suspended for fifty games for the infraction, Jacobs admitted to using the drug as part of an attempt to overcome knee and back problems. "Taking it was one of the worst decisions I could have ever made, one for which I take full responsibility,"[16] said Jacobs.

Blood Doping

While the fight against stimulants and steroids was producing results, the main front in the antidoping war was rapidly shifting to blood doping. There are a number of ways in which blood doping can take place: through blood transfusions, by injections of erythropoietin (EPO), and injections of synthetic oxygen carriers.

Blood transfusions, sometimes called "blood boosting," involve the removal and subsequent reinfusion of the athlete's blood to increase the level of oxygen-carrying hemoglobin. Blood transfusions have been used medically for decades to help patients who have lost blood due to injury or surgery, as well as for patients who have low red blood cell counts due to anemia, kidney failure, or other medical problems. In athletics, blood transfusions were first used to boost an athlete's performance in the 1970s. Some athletes draw their own blood and store it for future use (called autologous transfusion); others use the blood of someone else with the same blood type (homologous transfusion). Autologous transfusion is particularly difficult to detect because the athlete is using his or her own blood.

Gene Therapy and Doping

First conceptualized in 1972, gene therapy may be the latest medical advance to be adapted for the playing field. Essentially, gene therapy involves the manipulation and use of DNA as a pharmaceutical agent. Recent clinical tests have demonstrated the promise of gene therapy to treat a range of serious illnesses, but scientists worry about the risks of its use in otherwise healthy people.

Scientists have identified 187 genes linked to fitness and athleticism. Gene therapy could be used to build muscle, increase endurance, or otherwise boost performance. Ethicists are alarmed by the potential to use the life-saving therapy for sport. "In the gene therapy setting, we do these kinds of manipulations as a society, we accept [the risks] in the course of trying to do good and heal suffering—or heal illness and ease suffering," says Theodore Friedmann, the head of WADA's panel on gene doping. "But to do the same kinds of dangerous things to healthy young athletes is really unconscionable."

Talk of the Nation, "Experts: 'Gene Doping' to Be Next Sports Scandal," National Public Radio, February 5, 2010. www.npr.org.

Drug testers also have difficulty addressing methods of doping by which athletes artificially increase the production of red blood cells using the hormone EPO. EPO acts on stem cells in the bone marrow to increase the production of red blood cells, thereby increasing endurance. For many years the EPO ban could not be enforced due to the lack of a reliable testing method. In 2000 an EPO test was approved by WADA and began to be used at the Olympic Games that year in Sydney.

Another form of blood doping involves the use of synthetic oxygen carriers, which are purified proteins or chemicals that have the ability to carry oxygen just as human blood does. Synthetic oxygen carriers are useful for emergency situations in which human blood is not available or the risk of blood infection is high. The first test for synthetic oxygen carriers was implemented in 2004 at the Summer Olympic Games in Athens.

Oxygen doping dates back several decades but has seen a recent resurgence, perhaps as a result of the introduction of EPO detection methods. This suggests that as drug-testing methodology improves, athletes will continue to look for ways to beat the tests. "The history of sport tells us that there will be an ongoing struggle between athletes trying to bend/break the rules and drug testers trying to catch them," writes Chris Cooper in his 2012 book *Run, Swim, Throw, Cheat.* "Oxygen doping is not likely to escape. Apart from the obvious targets such as more EPO derivatives there are likely to be a panoply of compounds that will affect red cell development of which we are as yet unaware."[17]

"The history of sport tells us that there will be an ongoing struggle between athletes trying to bend/ break the rules and drug testers trying to catch them."[17]

— Chris Cooper, biochemist and author of *Run, Swim Throw, Cheat*.

Gene Doping

The most recent form of performance enhancement is a method called gene doping, which WADA defines as "the transfer of cells or genetic elements (e.g. DNA, RNA) [or] the use of pharmacological or biological agents that alter gene expression."[18] Gene doping builds on gene therapy, in which researchers have found ways to modify genes to prevent or treat serious medical conditions. The science of gene transfer makes it possible to put synthetic genes into human cells, where they become indistinguishable from a person's own DNA, the marker that defines a person's unique genetic makeup. This makes it possible for athletes and others to receive genes that can slow muscle deterioration, speed up the body's metabolism, or augment muscle performance.

The first product to be associated with gene doping emerged in 2006, when German authorities caught an athletic coach using the Internet to buy Repoxygen, a gene therapy material designed to produce EPO. Sports governing organizations believe that experts may begin to use the manipulation of genes to help athletes boost their performance. Although there are no known cases of gene doping, some experts say it is only a matter of time. Theodore Friedmann, the head of WADA's gene doping panel, warns that "with the improvement in the gene therapy technology, the extension to sport is becoming more and more inevitable."[19] According to the WADA website, "Gene doping represents a threat to the integrity of sport and the health of athletes."[20] To combat the threat, WADA has embarked on an ambitious program to identify ways to detect gene doping.

The Athlete Biological Passport

One new strategy for detecting advanced forms of doping involves something that WADA calls an athlete biological passport. A biological passport uses biological markers that provide a baseline for such things as red blood cell count and testosterone levels. Blood or urine samples taken from an athlete during competition can then be analyzed in comparison to an athlete's baseline measure. Variances between the established levels outside permissible limits are used to indicate that an athlete has used a banned substance. Advocates believe that the passport is an invaluable tool for detecting illegal use of substances that occur naturally in the human body, such as EPO, steroids, and human growth hormones.

The ICU used this method to test cyclists at the beginning of the 2008 season. Six cyclists received sanctions as the result of

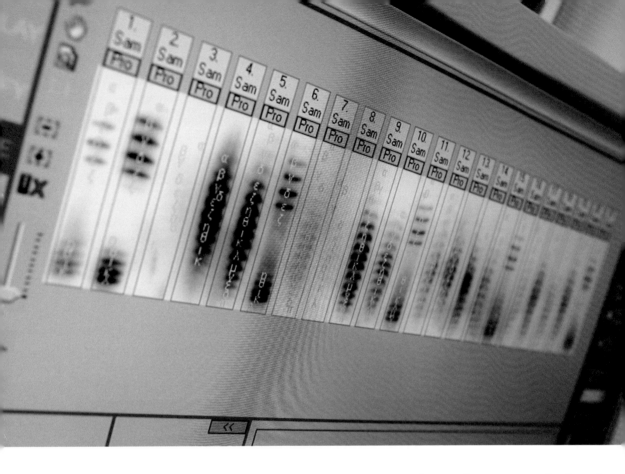

abnormalities detected in their biological passports, and several others were targeted for additional doping controls. A number of other athletic organizations, including IAFF and the IOC, have also begun drug testing that uses the athlete biological passport.

Past, Present, and Future

The authoritative body on the use of performance-enhancing drugs today is WADA, which oversees the testing of athletes for several sports federations and for the Olympic Games, which has the most aggressive drug-testing program in the world. As hawkers of performance-enhancing drugs improve the substances' sophistication, potency, and inability to be detected, WADA and its constituency work tirelessly to find new detection methods.

Today, more sports organizations are overseeing more drug-testing programs than ever before. More athletes than ever before, at all levels of competition and at ever younger ages, are given drug

A screen displays the results of a test for EPO, a hormone used by athletes to increase endurance by increasing the production of red blood cells. A reliable test for EPO did not exist until 2000.

tests, often conducted in conjunction with other drug-prevention efforts. Tests can detect more banned substances than ever before. Yet athletes at all levels continue to cheat, putting their reputations, their livelihoods, and their very lives at risk. "Doping continues to occur," concedes John Fahey, the president of WADA, "and it changes rapidly. There are athletes who are still lured by the glory of winning at all costs. And there are members of the athlete entourage still motivated to profit from an athlete's doping while risking little themselves. . . . The sad reality is there is still an enormous amount of work to be done."[21]

> "Doping continues to occur, and it changes rapidly. There are athletes who are still lured by the glory of winning at all costs. And there are members of the athlete entourage still motivated to profit from an athlete's doping while risking little themselves."[21]
>
> — John Fahey, president of the World Anti-Doping Agency.

Facts

- In 2011 the International Cycling Union (UCI) conducted a total of 7,900 urine and 5,244 blood tests (in-competition, pre-competition, and out-of-competition).

- The first full-scale testing of Olympic athletes began at the 1972 Summer Games, where 2,079 samples were analyzed. Seven athletes were disqualified after failing drug tests.

- There were no positive tests among the first 86 drug tests at the 1968 Winter Olympic Games. Of 667 drug tests performed at the 1968 Summer Olympic Games in Mexico City, one athlete (0.15 percent) tested positive.

- Weightlifting is the Olympic sport with the highest number of doping cases; between 1968 and 2010, thirty-six Olympic weightlifters failed drug tests. This is followed closely by track and field, with twenty-eight.

- The IOC conducted more than six thousand blood and urine tests during the 2012 Olympics; 9 athletes tested positive. An additional 117 athletes were caught cheating by antidoping agencies in the two months prior to competition.

- Major League Baseball (MLB) tests for HGH in the minor leagues, but clashes with the player's league about taking blood samples have prohibited it to test top players for the hormone.

- The HGH test currently used can detect synthetic growth hormone in someone's blood about thirty-six hours after the drug has been injected.

CHAPTER TWO

How Big a Problem Is Drug Use in Sports?

There is evidence that more athletes use performance-enhancing drugs than ever before. According to data from the World Anti-Doping Agency, there were fifteen thousand fewer drug tests in 2011 than in 2010, yet there were significantly more "adverse analytical findings" (positive tests). In fact, 2011 experienced the highest rate of positive drug tests since 2008. This is in part due to the fact that the tests have become more comprehensive, but it also illustrates that athletes continue to use performance-enhancing drugs.

Drug Use Fuels Testing in Professional Sports

In professional sports in the United States, the controversy over the use of performance-enhancing drugs dates back to the 1980s, when concerns were first raised about the use of steroids among football and baseball players, along with other professional athletes. Suspicions were heightened in the late 1990s, when sportswriters speculated openly about whether the race to beat the long-standing home-run record set by Roger Maris was fueled by steroids.

In 1998 Major League Baseball (MLB) players Sammy Sosa and Mark McGwire matched home run for home run, resulting in a record-breaking season in which both players outhit Maris's record. Both Sosa and McGwire denied using drugs to enhance their performance, but McGwire admitted he had taken andro-stenedione (a precursor to steroids that was not on the MLB list of banned drugs) to help him recover from an injury. In early 2010—more than a decade later—McGwire admitted that he had also used anabolic steroids. Although he apologized for his use of steroids, he reiterated that he began using steroids to heal from injury, not to improve his home run performance or batting average.

By the early 2000s there was growing evidence that the use of steroids and other performance-enhancing drugs was a problem among professional athletes. The players themselves began to admit that many colleagues were using drugs. In 2002 baseball player Ken Caminiti claimed that at least 50 percent of major league players used steroids. In his 2005 book *Juiced* Jose Canseco upped this figure to 85 percent.

MLB officials responded by instituting mandatory drug testing of players with severe penalties for those who broke the rules. As with the programs of the IOC, the program begins with a list of banned substances that includes steroids, stimulants, and illegal drugs. Testing is done through random drug testing conducted by an independent organization. On January 10, 2013, MLB and the players union reached an agreement to add random, in-season blood tests for HGH and baseline testosterone readings intended to help detect the use of testosterone.

> "Doping is cheating people out of their livelihood. If I go into a competition and somebody uses doping to beat me, they get my prize money."[23]
>
> — Andreas Thorkildsen, Olympic track and field athlete.

In addition to being the most aggressive testing programs among US professional sports programs, it also comes with the strictest penalties. Players who test positive for a banned substance receive a fifty-game suspension. A second positive test results in a one-hundred-game suspension, and players caught a third time receive a lifetime ban. Seven major league players were suspended for testing positive for performance-enhancing drugs in 2012, including All-Stars Marlon Byrd, Melky Cabrera, Bartolo Colon, and Carlos Ruiz. As of 2013 hitter Manny Ramirez and pitcher Guillermo Mota are the only two MLB players that have received one-hundred-game suspensions due to failing drug tests on two occasions.

Although MLB has been at the forefront of the controversy regarding performance-enhancing drugs, there is evidence of drug

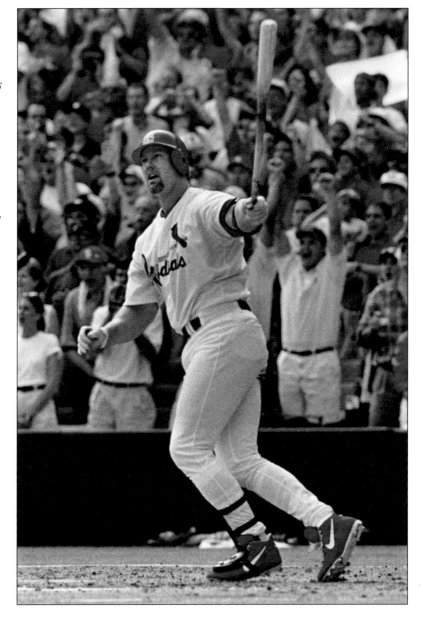

St. Louis Cardinals slugger Mark McGwire watches the ball sail over the left-field fence for his sixty-first home run of the 1998 season. More than a decade later McGwire admitted to using steroids, although he contended that he used them to heal from injury rather than to improve his game.

use in other sports as well. Some experts say that the sheer size of today's athletes is evidence of widespread steroid use. The average size of athletes in the National Football League (NFL), for instance, has increased significantly in the past two decades, and experts believe that steroids and human growth hormone are at the root of the change. Athletes at all levels are growing in size.

For instance, the average player on Michigan State University's football team in 1975 weighed 213 pounds (96.6 kg); the average weight in 2005 was 236 pounds (107 kg).

Confidential surveys of athletes themselves suggest extensive drug use. In 2009 nearly one in ten retired NFL players polled said they had used anabolic steroids while still playing. In 2010 Richard Pound, a Canadian member of the IOC and WADA, estimated that more than 30 percent of National Hockey League (NHL) players used performance-enhancing drugs.

With the accusations have come new drug-testing programs. The NFL began to test players for illegal drugs and anabolic steroids in 1987; today, the program has expanded to include random drug tests year round, and each player in the league is tested at least once a season. The NHL created its testing program in 2005, and individual random testing with no advance notice was introduced in 2013. The players' association has agreed to tests for steroids and illegal drugs but has squelched suggestions to add certain stimulants to the NHL's prohibited substance list.

Ensuring Fairness in Sport

One of the main reasons behind strict drug-testing policies is to ensure fairness and the integrity of competition. Proponents of drug tests say that sports fans want to be able to trust that the athletes are competing fairly and following the rules—rules that include a ban on performance-enhancing substances. John William Devine, a professor at New College in Oxford, writes, "We have reason to restrict the use of performance enhancing drugs in sport not only because of the threat they pose to athletes' health but also because of the threat they pose to athletes' displaying the relevant types of sporting excellence."[22]

Some athletes view the use of performance-enhancing drugs as a form of stealing. Andreas Thorkildsen, who won the Olympic Gold Medal in javelin in 2004 and 2008, says, "Doping is cheating people out of their livelihood. If I go into a competition and somebody uses doping to beat me, they get my prize money." Thorkildsen is among those who believe that there will always be cheaters in sports. "I'd like everyone to be clean, but as long as it is possible to cheat, someone will cheat,"[23] he says.

When one athlete cheats, others may feel they have to do so as well so that they are not at a disadvantage. Ellis Cashmore, a professor of culture, media, and sport at Staffordshire University in England who has conducted research into the use of drugs in sport, believes this is the main reason that athletes take drugs. "I don't think there's a conscious motivation when people dope to gain an unfair advantage," he explains. "My strong belief is that they are trying to level the playing field, knowing that there are so many others doping that they will be disadvantaged if they don't."[24] French cyclist Sebastien Hinault is among those who believes that tests are essential for ridding sport of doping: "In high level sport, cheating is part of the game," he writes in *Ouest-France*. "We will only be able to get rid of the cheats by multiplying testing."[25]

But not everyone agrees that drug testing is the answer. Some people argue that there will always be athletes that have access to the latest drugs and doctors who can help them beat the tests. Some people who follow this line of thinking believe that legalizing drugs in sport would be fairer. "Doping is not against the spirit of sport," says Julian Savulescu, an ethics professor at the Oxford Centre of Neuroethics. "It has always [been] part of the human spirit to use knowledge to make oneself better and doping has been a part of sport since its beginning."[26]

Proponents of legalizing performance-enhancing drugs say that they are no different from the diet, exercise, and other tools that an athlete uses to become bigger, stronger, faster, and/or more agile than the competition. In an article titled "Why We Should Allow Performance Enhancing Drugs in Sport," published in the *British Journal of Sports Medicine*, Savulescu, along with Bennett Foddy and M. Clayton of the Murdoch Childrens Research Institute, compare performance-enhancing drugs used by athletes to the drugs that classical musicians use to calm their nerves before a concert. "We should not think that allowing cyclists to take EPO would turn the Tour de France into some kind of 'drug race' any more than the various training methods available turn it into a 'training race' or a 'money race,'" the authors write. "Athletes train in different, creative ways, but ultimately they still ride similar bikes, on the same course. The skill of negotiating the steep winding descent will always be there."[27]

Yet another argument related to fairness involves the fact that different organizations have different drug-testing policies. This raises questions such as: Is it fair to test students at one college and not another? Does this give a school that does not have athlete drug-testing policies in place an unfair advantage? A related issue is the fact that some athletes may have better access to information than others. Top athletes have a team of doctors and trainers that can help them navigate the complexity of the drug-testing system to ensure that they can access the best supplements and dietary aids without unwittingly breaking the rules. At the international level, some national teams may have better access to such information than others.

Fairness issues may also arise when athletes are targeted for additional drug testing. In some cases, rather than being sanctioned for a first offense, an athlete who tests positive might be subject to ongoing drug testing. While often intended to allow athletes who may have inadvertently taken a banned (but not illegal) substance to continue to compete, some people believe the scrutiny puts them at a disadvantage—if only because it brings so much negative attention.

And so, the argument goes, we should ban only the substances that could clearly cause harm and allow those that are safe—at least at some dosage levels. Legalizing these substances would enhance safety by allowing them to be regulated. Rather than buying a steroid or HGH from the black market, for example, where the purity of the product is unknown, athletes could legally purchase performance-enhancing drugs made safer by regulation. "We allow people to do far more dangerous things than play football or baseball while using steroids," points out Norman Fost, a doctor who teaches medical ethics at the University of Wisconsin. "We allow people to bungee-jump, to ski on advanced slopes, to cliff dive. To eat marbled meat or ice cream pie every day if they

"In high level sport, cheating is part of the game. We will only be able to get rid of the cheats by multiplying testing."[25]

— French cyclist Sebastien Hinault.

31

want."[28] In fact, if performance-enhancing substances improve an athlete's strength, agility, or alertness, they may actually make a sport safer by reducing injuries.

Health Risks

Protecting the health of athletes is the other main argument for banning drugs and enforcing the bans with drug tests. Some experts argue that allowing any type of drugs by definition puts athletes' health at risk. Because everyone's body is different, one athlete might be able to withstand a high amount of a banned substance that would kill another person at much lower doses. "If doping were legal, it would be like asking athletes to place their health at risk just to compete at the same level as those already doping," argues the Ministry of Sport in Quebec, Canada. Richard Pound, the former president of WADA, suggests that athletes could become embroiled in a race in which they are encouraged to take drugs at an ever increasing—and ever more dangerous—dosage: "Remember that athletes don't take these drugs to level the playing field, they do it to get an advantage. And if everyone else is doing what they're doing, then instead of taking 10 grams or 10 cc's or whatever it is, they'll take 20 or 30 or 40, and a vicious circle simply gets bigger. The end game will be an activity that is increasingly violent, extreme, and meaningless, practiced by a class of chemical and or genetic mutant gladiators."[29]

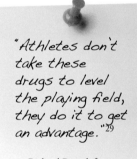

Thomas H. Murray, president of the Hastings Center, an independent think tank focused on bioethics, agrees. "Sports that revere records and historical comparisons (think of baseball and home runs) would become unmoored by drug-aided athletes obliterating old standards," he writes. "Athletes, caught in the sport arms race, would be pressed to take more and more drugs, in ever wilder combinations and at increasingly higher doses. The drug race in sport has the potential to create a slow-motion public health catastrophe."[30]

One does not need to look very far to find examples of athletes who have sacrificed their health in the quest for glory. The wide-

The BALCO Incident

In 2003 the USADA received an anonymous call that a number of athletes were using tetrahydrogestrinone (THG), a designer steroid that users had nicknamed "the clear" because it could not be detected in drug tests. Federal agents raided the Burlingame, California, facility of the Bay Area Laboratory Co-operative (BALCO), the alleged manufacturer of the drug. In addition to evidence of steroids and growth hormones, the agents found a list of BALCO customers. Among them were several prominent MLB payers, NFL players, and Olympic athletes.

The BALCO incident highlighted the widespread use of performance-enhancement drugs among elite athletes and sparked a congressional investigation into the use of steroids. In the resulting report, Congress detailed a deep-rooted drug culture within Major League Baseball and listed eighty-nine players suspected of using performance-enhancing drugs. As players were called to testify before Congress, many found themselves in a swirl of media attention that focused not on their accomplishments but on their character. The experience was a wake-up call for MLB, which set about strengthening its drug-testing policies, and for a number of individual athletes who suddenly found themselves vilified as dopers, cheaters, and liars.

spread steroid use among East German Olympic athletes in the 1980s led to long-term health problems that continue to plague the athletes today. The women on the East German swimming team have had an abnormal number of issues related to infertility and miscarriages attributed to the use of steroids, which several of the women say were given to them without their knowledge.

Perhaps the most public face of the steroid scandal is Heidi Krieger, a female shot-putter who was given so many steroids that she later opted to have a sex change and is today known as Andreas. Anabolic steroids are especially dangerous for females because the female body is not equipped to manage large doses of the hormone. Males produce about twenty to thirty times as much testosterone as females do.

Any athlete can be at risk. In expert testimony before Congress, sports medicine expert Linn Goldberg, who has led studies on performance-enhancing drugs for the Oregon Health & Science University in Portland, testified that high levels of HGH can cause acromegaly, a degenerative disease characterized by extreme swelling of the limbs and joint pains. Goldberg warned Congress that the disease increased the risk of "diabetes, high blood pressure, and premature cardiovascular disease. Over years, peripheral nerve damage and muscle weakening can occur."[31]

There are many cases in which drug use is assumed to be a contributing factor to premature death among athletes in a variety of sports at many different levels. Baltimore Orioles pitcher Steve Bechler died of heatstroke at the age of twenty-three; post-autopsy reports blamed a supplement called ephedra that he was taking in

Russian ice hockey player Alexei Cherepanov and teammates celebrate a goal in 2007. The following year, Cherepanov, 19, collapsed and died during a game. Tests revealed he had been blood doping.

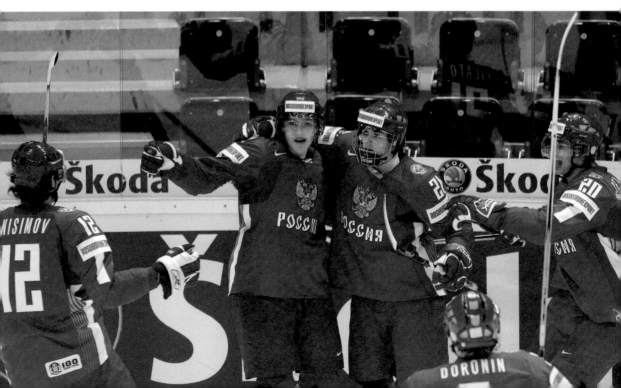

an effort to lose weight. During a 2008 game in Russia's Continental Hockey League, Alexei Cherepanov, a prospect for the National Hockey League's New York Rangers, collapsed on the bench and died. Russian federal investigators ruled that Cherepanov, who reportedly died of a heart condition, had been blood doping. He was just nineteen years old.

Performance-Enhancing Drugs and Teens

One of the main concerns about allowing elite athletes to use performance-enhancing drugs is that it would not only put their lives at risk but also encourage the use of drugs among young people. "As is often the case, the high school student-athletes are modeling this illicit behavior of drug use by professional and college athletes," writes Robert A. Stinchcomb. "It is this level of competition that raises so many questions."[32]

If drugs are dangerous for adult athletes in prime condition, they are infinitely more so for people whose brains and bodies are still growing. Taking drugs during or before adolescence can have permanent consequences. Animal studies undertaken at the Geisel School of Medicine at Dartmouth College, for instance, show a relationship between the use of anabolic steroids during adolescence and lifelong depression, aggression, and sexual dysfunction, as well as cancer and liver disease. Anabolic steroids increase aggression and have been blamed for everything from poor performance in school to road rage to homicide. Among the most widely publicized examples was Taylor Hooton, a high school baseball player who began taking anabolic steroids at sixteen to gain size and strength. On July 15, 2003, at the age of seventeen, Hooton committed suicide, an act that his parents insist was related to the steroids.

In the Youth Risk Behavior Surveillance summary of 2011, 3.6 percent of students reported that they had taken steroid pills or shots without a doctor's prescription one or more times during their life. Although this means that half a million students have taken steroids, the same study found that steroid use had decreased since 2003, when it reached 6.1 percent. Experts worry that other performance-enhancing drugs such as HGH may be replacing steroids.

Caffeine: To Ban or Not to Ban

Caffeine is a stimulant that has long been used by athletes to improve alertness and concentration. Caffeine has been shown to improve performance in any event that requires exercise for over five minutes. According to biochemist Chris Cooper, "when it comes to running or cycling, caffeine can increase the time to exhaustion by as much as twenty to fifty percent." Cooper goes on to explain the on-again/off-again approach to banning caffeine:

"This does rather beg the question why caffeine is not banned. Indeed at first caffeine use was made a doping offence, though somewhat bizarrely the levels that resulted in a ban were higher than those considered to be performance enhancing. However, since 2004 this ban has been lifted; it is now fine to have a coffee before you run—at least if you are a human. It is still banned in racehorses. The rationale here, one assumes, is that caffeine is considered a normal part of a human diet, but horses don't usually hang out at Starbucks. Recently, the introduction of caffeine pills by athletes has led to concerns about whether to reintroduce a ban. Although these pills are no more effective than drinking two or three very strong espressos at raising caffeine levels, the negative perception of taking a pill seems to be the concern. Speaking in July 2010 John Fahey, the president of the World Anti-Doping Agency, said that taking pills is against the spirit of sport."

Chris Cooper, *Run, Swim, Throw, Cheat: The Science Behind Drugs in Sport*. Oxford, UK: Oxford University Press, 2012, page 176.

Nora D. Volkow, the director of the National Institute on Drug Abuse, emphasizes that anabolic steroids may present a far greater risk for young people than illegal street drugs:

Abuse of anabolic steroids differs from the abuse of other

illicit substances because the initial abuse of anabolic steroids is not driven by the immediate euphoria that accompanies most drugs of abuse, such as cocaine, heroin, and marijuana, but by the desire of abusers to change their appearance and performance, characteristics of great importance to adolescents. The effects of steroids can boost confidence and strength, leading abusers to overlook the potential serious and long-term damage that these substances can cause.[33]

Leaders of the Taylor Hooton Foundation, which was created in honor of Hooton, agree with Volkow's assessment. "Young people today are under tremendous amounts of pressure," warns its website. "The desire to win, to look good, to earn a scholarship can create insurmountable stress. This pressure comes from peers, teachers, coaches, and even parents. The desire to succeed at any cost can force a student or athlete to make a deadly mistake."[34]

Putting an end to the risks for teens requires putting an end to the use of performance-enhancing drugs among teens' athletic heroes and role models. To this end, the goal of drug testing would not be to catch athletes who have used the drugs but rather to provide an incentive for avoiding the drugs altogether. Whether this is a realistic goal remains to be seen.

> "The effects of steroids can boost confidence and strength, leading abusers to overlook the potential serious and long-term damage that these substances can cause."[33]
>
> — Nora D. Volkow, director of the National Institute on Drug Abuse.

Facts

- Studies have shown that the transfusion of half a liter of blood can increase the capacity of muscles to use oxygen by up to 5 percent.

- Studies involving the anabolic steroid androgen show that, even in doses much lower than those used by athletes, muscular strength can be improved by 5 to 20 percent.

- National Football League testing reported twenty-one tests positive for performance-enhancing drugs in 2012, a 75 percent increase over 2011. Some believe the increase to be due to the addition of tests for prescription medications for ADHD.

- The Mayo Clinic estimates that twenty European cyclists have died as a result of blood doping over the past twenty-five years.

- The Taylor Hooton Foundation reports that the median age that a teen first uses anabolic steroids is fifteen.

- According to a June 2013 report by ESPN's "Outside the Lines" investigative team, MLB planned to initiate suspension proceedings against approximately twenty baseball players in what could become the largest PED scandal in the history of US sports. The players were alleged to have links to a now-closed clinic in Florida that has been the focus of an MLB investigation into PED use. ESPN reported that players charged with more than one offense could face one hundred-game suspensions.

CHAPTER THREE

How Fair and Reliable Are Drug-Testing Methods and Policies?

Different sports organizations apply different restrictions and testing procedures to stop the use of performance-enhancing drugs, with varying rates of success. The most vigorous drug-testing program is overseen by WADA for the IOC, and other organizations often base their list of banned substances and the methods for detection on Olympic standards. The intent of these programs is to catch and sanction athletes who cheat, thereby increasing the fairness of the competition and the integrity of the sport. Colleges and high schools often have a different reason for drug testing: to deter young people from using illegal drugs and get help for those who test positive before they become victims of drug use.

The List

WADA's list of banned substances and methods has become the standard used by more than six hundred athletic federations worldwide. The list is long—outlining roughly two hundred different substances and methods that are prohibited. The classes of prohibited substances include anabolic agents (steroids); hormones and related substances; beta-2 agonists, a class of drugs developed to treat asthma and pulmonary diseases; hormone antagonists and modulators, which are messenger molecules that regulate blood sugar levels, muscle growth, and other specific body functions; stimulants; narcotics; and diuretics and other masking agents. The list also includes banned methods such as blood doping and gene doping, as well as tampering with samples.

WADA reviews the list annually, adding or removing drugs as warranted. Although the list names specific drugs, it comes with a warning for athletes that the list of prohibited substances is not intended to be comprehensive. "A key concept in prohibited lists is that they avoid being finite," explains Caroline Hatton, a sports antidoping science consultant. "Instead of listing all banned drugs one by one, they list entire drug classes and name drugs merely as examples. This is to keep users who took designer drugs from claiming that they didn't break the rules because the drugs they took weren't listed."[35]

It is this lack of clarity that troubles some athletes. Athletes worry that they will test positive for a banned substance ingested unwittingly. Some athletes worry that a positive drug test could result from eating food with an opiate, such as a poppy-seed bagel or muffin, or meat from an animal that has been injected with hormones. Athletes also complain that it is impossible to "vet" vitamins, protein powders, and other dietary supplements to ensure that they do not include anything on the banned substance list.

Some athletes have argued that the only way they can know for sure that nothing in their diet of supplements will lead to a positive result is to allow them to take a confidential drug test ahead of time. Accredited laboratories are prohibited from conducting tests unless authorized as part of an athletic organization's drug program, however. Experts who run the drug-testing programs say there is good reason for these requirements, as it keeps the laboratories from either intentionally or inadvertently helping athletes who want to

"There are many drugs doctors are legally permitted to administer to Tour de France riders. Why are some approved and others not?"[37]

— Jonathan Mahler, sports columnist.

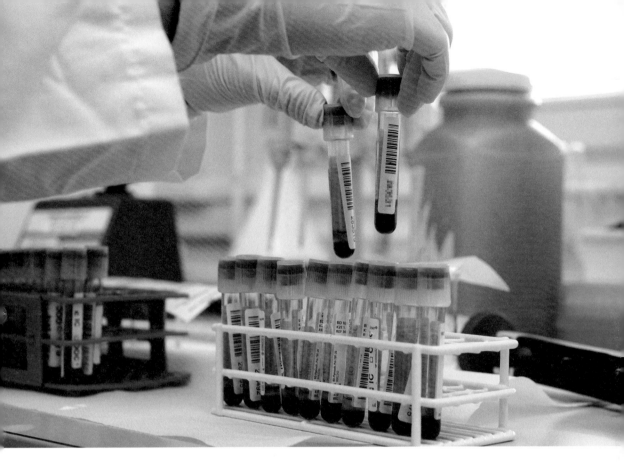

learn how to evade detection. In 2010 a message string at a triathlon forum was begun by someone asking whether there was a way to run a "preemptive" drug test. "MBannon" responded, "This is an interesting topic, especially as WADA's (and presumably USADA's) stance is that athletes are responsible for knowing what they are putting into their bodies. Yet there is no way to test this stuff."[36]

Who Decides?

One of the criticisms about drug testing is that it includes substances that are legal in other settings. Critics raise questions about who decides which substances are banned and on what grounds the decisions are made. "There are many drugs doctors are legally permitted to administer to Tour de France riders. Why are some approved and others not?" asks sports columnist Jonathan Mahler in an article following Armstrong's confession that he used drugs. "Why does cortisone—which alleviates pain and enhances

A Swiss doping analysis laboratory technician prepares blood to be tested for human growth hormone and blood transfusion. Sports organizations use a variety of testing procedures, some more reliable than others.

performance—represent an acceptable level of pharmaceutical aid, but not, say, stanozolol?"[37]

Critics also call into question some of the decisions about drugs that can be taken with a doctor's prescription, claiming that if these drugs are safe for someone who is ill to take, they should be safe enough to be taken by the world's healthiest athletes who are under the constant care of physicians. The athlete's physician, these critics say, not drug-testing organizations, should be the one to decide whether he or she would benefit from a painkiller, sleeping aid, or other medication.

On the other side of the argument are those who believe that physicians are not necessarily concerned about an athlete's health or the long-term consequences of performance-enhancing drug use. Some athletes caught taking banned substances say they were following the advice or instructions of doctor or trainer. US track and field star Marion Jones, who was later stripped of her Olympic medals after failing drug tests, says her coach gave her THG for several months before she even knew what it was for. "He told me to put it under my tongue for a few seconds and swallow it," she said. "He told me not to tell anyone."[38] George Mavrotas, a commissioner of Greece's Olympic committee, says that even when they know what they are doing, "The doped athlete is not an innocent victim, but he is a victim after all. . . . [The cheater] bears the consequences while the true responsible (coaches, managers, doctors, etc.) usually remain unpunished and continue this business."[39]

> "The doped athlete is not an innocent victim, but he is a victim after all. . . . [The cheater] bears the consequences while the true responsible (coaches, managers, doctors, etc.) usually remain unpunished and continue this business."[39]
>
> — George Mavrotas, a commissioner of Greece's Olympic committee.

Inadvertent Use of Banned Substances

Many of the drugs on the list of banned substances are available over-the-counter or with a prescription, and athletes with a positive drug test are quick to claim that they did not realize a prescription or over-the-counter drug had an ingredient on the list of banned drugs. Athletes may make this claim as a cover-up for intended drug use, but there are also clearly instances in which the use of banned substances is inadvertent.

Banned Substances

There are hundreds of substances that can affect an athlete's performance. Not all of them are prohibited by athletic organizers. Some of the substances, like caffeine, are found in many different types of food and have no restrictions. Others, like cortisone or narcotic painkillers, are allowable with a doctor's prescription if an athlete is recovering from an injury. WADA lists twelve categories of banned substances and methods:

- Anabolic agents, including anabolic androgenic steroids and other anabolic agents such as clenbuterol
- Hormones and related substances, including erythropoietin (EPO), human growth hormone (hGH), gonadotrophins, insulins, and corticotophins
- Beta-2 agonists, used to treat asthma and other pulmonary diseases
- Hormone antagonists and modulators, which encourage or discourage the release of hormones
- Diuretics and other masking agents
- Stimulants, including illegal drugs such as cocaine, prescription drugs such as Adderall, and over-the-counter medications used to remedy cold symptoms
- Narcotics, including opiates and other painkillers
- Cannabinoids (marijuana and hashish)
- Glucocorticosteroids, which are anti-inflammatory agents
- Alcohol
- Beta-Blockers, used to treat anxiety and high blood pressure
- Banned methods, including blood doping, chemical and physical manipulation of drug-testing samples, and gene doping

Romanian gymnast Andrea Raducan, for example, was stripped of the gold and silver medals she won at the 2000 Olympic Games in Sydney after testing positive for pseudoephedrine, an ingredient in a decongestant that she had taken for a cold. Olga Medvedtseva, an Olympic biathlete from Russia, failed a drug test in 2006 after carphedon, a stimulant, was found in her system. The Russian Anti-Doping Committee explained that she tested positive for the stimulant because she was given an over-the-counter drug to treat an ankle injury. The manufacturer did not have a complete list of the compounds in the drug she used. Although the failed drug test was not Medvedtseva's fault, she was issued a two-year suspension. She returned to the sport to win a gold medal at the 2010 Olympic Games in Vancouver.

Sometimes an athlete is stripped of an Olympic medal after testing positive and/or admitting to drug use many years later. Marion Jones's admission to steroid use had a profound impact on her past teammates. In 2008 the IOC ruled that eight women involved in running relay races with Jones also had to return their medals. The women filed an appeal with the Court of Arbitration for Sport. "We are being unfairly punished," argued Chryste Gaines, who ran with Jones in the 2000 Olympic Games. "If the drug testing agencies cannot determine if an athlete is taking performance enhancing drugs how are the teammates supposed to know?"[40]

There have also been instances in which athletes have tested positive for drugs that they have been prescribed for a medical condition. Most regulatory organizations allow players to get waivers to use prescription drugs for medical purposes, but some players may neglect to complete the necessary paperwork. This appears to be what happened to Will Hill, a safety with the New York Giants who received a four-game suspension from the NFL after testing positive for Adderall, a common drug used to treat attention deficit/hyperactivity disorder (ADHD). Hill had a prescription for the drug, which he had begun using in high school to treat the symptoms of ADHD. He was using the drug before signing with the Giants. He knew that Adderall was among the substances banned by the NFL but reportedly was unaware that he could get a waiver.

Other challenges involve seemingly innocent prescription and over-the-counter drugs that are used by athletes not to enhance performance but for the same reasons that they benefit nonathletes. Under the parameters of drug-testing programs, athletes are unable to take stimulants to stay awake for a long drive, or sleeping remedies like Ambien that might help them calm down after a big game or deal with changes in time zones. Athletes might also worry about taking a drug to address symptoms of a common cold, flu, or other illness. Because such substances can potentially be used as a performance-enhancing drug, they are off-limits to athletes for any purpose.

Urine and Blood Tests

Once the list of banned substances has been determined, the rules are enforced through drug testing. The most widely used drug tests rely on urine samples. The reliability of a urine test requires ensuring that it is the athlete who is providing the sample and that there is no way for the sample to be contaminated between the time it is taken and when it is analyzed. The most reliable drug tests are conducted randomly so that the athlete has no way to prepare for the test or neutralize a drug's effects through masking agents. Many drugs do not stay in the system for long. The purpose of drug testing is to ensure that athletes remain clean, not that they avoid drugs the week that the drug tests are being conducted.

Some banned substances, including HGH, cannot be detected in an athlete's urine. To detect these substances requires a blood sample. Blood testing has been used by several athletic federations, including the IOC and the UCI, for many years. In 2012 the NFL became the first American sports league to carry out blood testing at the major professional league level.

In some cases, blood tests are conducted only when an athlete is suspected of utilizing blood doping. Because blood tests are expensive and have met with considerable opposition by some athletes, some sports organizations have looked for needles or other evidence before ordering a blood test. Some sports federations have sought for leeway to search the homes or lockers of athletes for such evidence, but many people believe that inspections are a clear violation of an athlete's privacy.

Random and Targeted Tests

Essentially, athletic organizations use two types of drug tests: random and targeted. Generally, random drug tests select a name from a pool of athletes; how large this pool is and the athlete's likelihood of being selected for drug testing varies greatly depending on the sport and its governing federation. Targeted testing, which is done by the IOC, tests top athletes in sports that have a history of drug use. While universal testing that would test all athletes for drugs might be preferable, the cost of testing every athlete is prohibitive. Moreover, a program that schedules all athletes for drug tests on any given day is generally ineffective because athletes are on notice, so they can schedule their drug use accordingly. Even so, there is no such thing as totally random testing. "It's not really random at all," says Travis Tygart, the head of the USADA. "We concentrate both our testing numbers as well as our special analysis at the high-risk sports and the high-risk athletes."[41]

World champion shot-putter Christian Cantwell has been tested at least 104 times between 2001 and 2012, among the highest numbers for a US athlete. Cantwell has never tested positive for drug use, but he worries that he will be banned anyway. Cantwell recently missed a surprise test when a testing official showed up at his house in Missouri while Cantwell was at a competition in Boston. Even though he was tested at the competition, Cantwell's missed test counts the same as if he had tested positive. "A guy like me, who's completely clean, has nothing to hide. . . . They can still give me a ban for missed tests," complains Cantwell. "It's absurd."[42]

Keeping Athletes on Notice

The strictest drug-testing programs test athletes not only before and immediately after competition but also during the off-season. This is because some drugs, such as anabolic steroids, have an effect long after they are taken.

There are considerable obstacles to testing athletes off-season, however. Athletes often travel a lot and can be difficult to find. Notification can also be difficult. Some cheaters were ensuring that they could not be notified of a test by filling up their cell phones with other messages so that a message from an official tester could not get through. In 2012 the IOC adopted new notification procedures that require Olympic athletes to notify the committee of where one will be one hour each day, 365 days a year, including holidays, during competition, and on travel days.

Several athletes say the rules are confusing and that there are days in anyone's life when it is almost impossible to know ahead of time where one would be. Olympic discus champion Stephanie Brown Trafton, who missed a test because she was out walking her dogs when a testing agent showed up at her house, is worried that she'll accidentally miss another. "I feel like I can't go anywhere or do anything without this fear of being caught for a missed test," she says. "And I'm not the one they're looking for, basically, because I test clean every single time."[43]

However, some athletes claim that the new system is easy to follow. Most of the tracking is done online, and an athlete can change his or her location and/or the hour that they will be available for testing. Lisa Galaviz, a member of the US steeplechase team, says, "I find it much easier to give one hour every day that I'll be home, rather than trying to designate where I am all the time."[44] Swiss tennis player Roger Federer believes that the new notification rules will help catch cheaters: "This is how you're going to catch them, right? You're not going to catch them ringing them up and saying, 'Look, I would like to test you maybe in two days.' The guy's cheating and they're smart, right? It's an hour a day. I know it's a pain, but I would like it to be a clean sport, and that's why I'm OK with it."[45]

> "I feel like I can't go anywhere or do anything without this fear of being caught for a missed test. And I'm not the one they're looking for, basically, because I test clean every single time."[43]
>
> — Stephanie Brown Trafton, Olympic discus athlete.

The Appeals Process

Almost all amateur and professional sports organizations allow an athlete to appeal a positive drug test, and the appeals are sometimes successful. One example was the case of British skier Alain

Baxter, who was stripped of the bronze medal he won at the 2002 Olympic Games in Salt Lake City after testing positive for traces of a methamphetamine. Baxter claimed that he did not realize that the ingredients of the Vicks inhaler he had used were different in the United States from those in Great Britain. The IOC accepted his explanation and reduced his two-year suspension to just three months; an appeal undertaken on Baxter's behalf by the British Ski and Snowboard Federation overturned the ban, but a separate appeal to have his medal returned to him was unsuccessful.

Professional athletes have also successfully appealed sanctions. In February 2012, Milwaukee Brewers player Ryan Braun, who earned the National League's award for Most Valuable Player in 2011, became the first MLB player to successfully appeal a positive drug test. Braun's positive test was due to unusually high levels of testosterone, often an indication of steroid use. He was slammed with a fifty-game suspension. The panel that heard Braun's appeal voted 2-1 to revoke the suspension after hearing evidence that the test collector had taken the urine sample home and stored it in his refrigerator for two days before shipping it to a testing laboratory. Although this was within the standard procedure specified by MLB, it raised questions among those who believed that it took too long to get the sample to the laboratory, which proved to be sufficient for the panel hearing Braun's appeal to overturn the decision to suspend him for testing positive.

Athletes who take common over-the-counter drugs for symptoms of cold, flu, or other illness risk positive drug tests and penalties even when they are not using these drugs to gain the advantage over their competition.

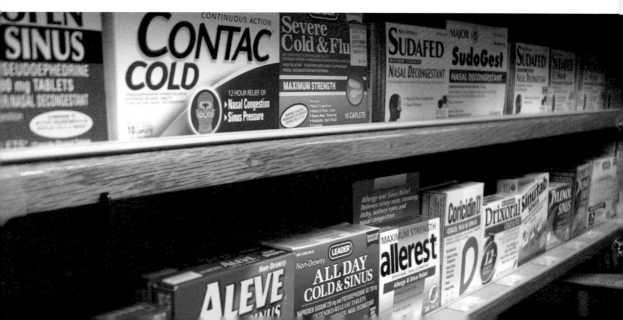

While some said that Braun's case cast doubt on the integrity of the drug-testing process, others stood by the drug tests. "You're not going to grow synthetic testosterone just because it sat in a refrigerator over the weekend," says Travis T. Tygart, the chief executive of the United States Anti-Doping Agency. "It's the best practice that when you can't get it to the lab because it's a weekend to keep it in the possession of the person who's trained to handle it, the doping control officer."[46] In a separate interview, Tygart laments the review panel's finding: "To have this sort of technicality of all technicalities let a player off . . . it's just a sad day for all the clean players and those that abide by the rules within professional baseball."[47]

Faking Out the Tests

Anyone who surfs the Internet will find a plethora of websites that claim athletes can fake out a test if needed. Some people have been duped into buying a product that will supposedly cleanse, detox, or purify the system so the drug test will come out negative. There also have been claims of athletes who have brought in "clean" urine samples to a testing facility or managed to dilute the sample with water or add bleach or another purification substance.

Experts say that none of these systems work. The claims of most so-called detox products are simply bogus, and laboratories test for diuretics or other masking agents that may actually work. In addition, the drug-testing process includes strict protocols to eliminate any possibility of switching the sample with another or tampering with the sample. Unlike drug tests used in an employment setting, the testing protocols for elite athletes usually include observing as the athlete provides the sample. The process also ensures that athletes notified to take a drug test cannot get out of it by simply not showing up; in most cases, a no-show or other act of noncompliance is considered to be a positive test.

Validity and Reliability

In appeals, athletes have questioned the validity of drug tests, claiming that a positive sample has been misidentified, improperly stored, or incorrectly tested. Athletes also have raised the possibility of sabotage of a urine sample, but there have been no confirmed cases of this occurring at any level of athletics. To combat such criticisms, testing facilities have a strict and well-documented chain of custody. The process usually involves having the athlete oversee the sample from the time it is collected to when it is sealed and labeled.

At the testing laboratory, strict protocols continue to ensure the integrity of the results. Upon arrival of a sample, a laboratory employee signs for it and checks to ensure that it is sealed properly. Another employee signs when the seal is broken. At each stage of the process, a laboratory technician validates that the sample has not been tampered with. This chain of custody helps ensure the accuracy of the results. Pathologist Anthony Butch, the director of the UCLA Olympic Analytical Laboratory, which is WADA's largest, emphasizes its importance. "All the appeals I've been to [athletes] debate the chain of command," he says. "The science is pretty hard to argue."[48]

The Science Behind the Tests

Still, experts agree that some substances are harder to detect than others. Banned substances like cocaine or artificial steroids that are not found naturally in the body are relatively easy to deal with, but some banned substances may exist naturally, albeit in small quantities. This adds to the complexity of the testing process. Nandrolone is an example.

A close chemical cousin of testosterone, nandrolone was thought to exist only in laboratories until a 2009 study showed that people can naturally have a small but significant level in their bodies. The highest level that has ever been detected is 0.6 nanograms per milliliter of urine, causing the IOC to set a limit of 2.0 nanograms per milliliter. Critics say that in cases like this, setting a limit for the maximum amount of these substances that would presumably be found naturally opens the door for an innocent athlete to test positive, particularly given the fact that the unusual stresses on an athlete's body during competition could raise the natural levels of a testosterone-like substance. Even those within the drug-testing environment have admitted that there are gray areas. "Things are so complex now that it's very hard to make it

Drug Testing at the Olympics

The International Olympic Committee has led the way in banning performance-enhancing drugs and in implementing strict drug-testing policies to enforce its zero-tolerance policy. The program aims for the protection of the health of athletes, respect for medical and sports ethics, and equality for all athletes. "The fight against doping is the number one priority for the IOC," reads an IOC fact sheet. "It is a question of ethics and health, linked to the Fundamental Principles of the Olympic Movement, such as fair play."

An independent medical commission is responsible for overseeing the IOC's drug-testing program, which combines mandatory and random drug-testing methodology. At Olympic events, the top five finishers in each event are tested, plus another two whose names are drawn out of the testing pool list. The tests are conducted immediately after the event, usually within ninety minutes.

In addition, there is random, unannounced year-round testing of Olympic athletes. Rules enacted in 2012 require athletes on Olympic teams to provide the IOC with a schedule of where they will be for one hour each day. Some athletes say the notification rules are cumbersome, but others believe they are necessary to keep the Olympics free of doping.

International Olympic Committee, "Factsheet: The Fight Against Doping and the Promotion of Athletes' Health," January 2010. http://sportsanddrugs.procon.org.

perfect,"[49] concedes Don Catlin, the founder and former director of the UCLA laboratory.

Blood doping is particularly difficult to test for, particularly when it involves an athlete's own blood. Tests usually involve identifying a person's hematocrit (HCT), which is the fraction of blood by volume occupied by red blood cells, and the concentration of hemoglobin. An HCT count between 41 to 50 percent is considered normal in adult men and 36 to 44 percent in women; normal hemoglobin levels are 14 to 17 grams per deciliter of blood in men and 12 to 15 grams per deciliter in women. Higher concentrations suggest an abnormally high level of red blood cells, which is often evidence of blood doping. The percentage of reticulocytes, immature red blood cells, can also point to blood doping.

In all of these instances, detecting blood doping often requires comparison of an athlete's blood over time. In 2009 Claudia Pechstein, a German speed skater and five-time Olympic gold medalist, became one of the first athletes to be sanctioned for alleged blood doping after tests revealed that she consistently had higher percentages of reticulocytes in her blood during competitions than at other times.

As with the nandrolone example, however, unusually high concentrations of red blood cells could be a naturally occurring medical condition. Critics of drug tests worry that this could result in a positive test for blood doping. Athletes are often required to keep a record of their blood test results as evidence of their innocence—a process that seems to assume that athletes are guilty unless proven innocent and puts the burden of proof on the athlete. The new athletic biological passport is part of the process that is intended to clarify gray areas and ensure that athletes with unusually high levels of red blood cells or other genetic anomalies will not be penalized.

A relatively new phenomenon, drug testing is an imperfect science. Drug-testing organizations have employed some of the world's top scientists to develop new tests for new performance-enhancing substances. Sports-governing organizations do not employ a new test until they are sure that it is accurate and fair to athletes. Procedures are designed to ensure the integrity of the testing. Still, there is always a risk of false positives. The appeals process is intended to provide a means for addressing these unusual incidents, but it too is imperfect. Still, most experts and clean athletes agree that sports are fairer with drug testing than without.

Facts

- The NFL conducts roughly 14,000 tests on 2,500 players each year.

- In 2010, the last year for which there is officially published data, WADA executed testing on 180,584 urine and blood serum samples taken from athletes in Olympic sports and 77,683 in non-Olympic sports.

- Experts estimate that the annual cost of WADA-related drug testing for Olympic and other elite amateur athletes is over $40 million.

- As of 2010 there are 625 organizations worldwide that used WADA's code that lists banned performance-enhancing substances and methods.

- In a 2009 survey of college athletes undertaken by the National Collegiate Athletic Association (NCAA), almost 60 percent of the respondents indicated that they strongly agree or agree that all college athletes should be drug tested by their school and/or the NCAA.

- Most college athletes are relatively unlikely to be tested for drug use. The International Amateur Athletic Federation estimates that only 10 to 15 percent of participating athletes are tested in each major competition.

- Most athletic organizations rely on WADA-certified laboratories for drug test analysis; as of 2013 WADA had thirty-five laboratories in thirty-two countries worldwide.

CHAPTER FOUR

What Role Should Drug Testing Play in Student Athletics?

I n the 1995 landmark case *Vernonia School District 47J v. Acton*, the Supreme Court ruled 6-3 that drug testing of interscholastic athletes was constitutional. The court rejected a claim asserting that such tests are protected by the privacy provisions of the Fourth Amendment to the Constitution. The ruling moved the debate regarding athlete drug testing from professional league ballparks and Olympic venues to the playgrounds and playing fields of the nation's schools.

Drug Testing at the Collegiate Level

Widespread drug testing of athletes at the collegiate level began in the late 1980s, after the National Collegiate Athletic Association (NCAA) voted at its 1986 annual convention to start a drug-testing program. Since then, the NCAA has been aggressive about encouraging the use of drug testing for college athletes, particularly those at highest levels of competition. Some top NCAA players are subject to random testing with forty-eight hours' notice and are randomly tested throughout the annual bowl game season. The NCAA does not publicly disclose a complete list of its banned substances but does release information on eight broad classes of banned drugs that might be tested for. Each test includes screening for at least one performance-enhancing drug. Andrea Wickerham, vice president of the Drug Free Sport testing organization, defends the NCAA practice of listing classes of banned drugs rather than a specific list of these drugs. She explains that the menu of banned drugs is "changing practically daily."[50]

Beyond the NCAA program, individual colleges, universities, high schools, and even middle schools are beginning to implement their own antidoping and drug-testing programs. The majority of universities with athletes at the highest competitive level (Division I) have drug-testing programs beyond what the NCAA requires.

Like Olympic athletes, student athletes at the most competitive-level schools have become used to drug testing. The NCAA and participating schools follow the protocol established by elite athletic organizations. For most student athletes the entire process—from the beginning through sealing the box in which the sample is placed—takes about fifteen minutes. (It may take longer following a competition when athletes are dehydrated and struggle to provide an adequate sample.) Brian Hendrickson, a journalist who went through the process to see how it worked, writes, "By the time it was done, I realized it wasn't a big deal. And from what I soon learned, most NCAA student-athletes feel the same way about the testing process. For those involved, it's merely a routine procedure with little drama."[51]

One of the issues involved in athlete drug testing at schools is that the drug tests sometimes focus on substances other than performance-enhancing substances. At the University of Oregon, for instance, the drug-testing program was stepped up after a 2012 report in *ESPN* magazine revealed that 40 to 60 percent of the football team at the school smoked marijuana. The university's drug policy allowed for testing when there was reasonable suspicion; the university used the *ESPN* report as evidence that a more aggressive drug-testing policy was needed and began to implement random drug tests.

High School Programs

The use of drugs among high school students has led to athlete drug-testing programs being proposed and implemented at this level of competition as well. A 2012 study found that about 5 percent of middle and high school students have used anabolic steroids to put on muscle, which critics blame on the pressure to look good as well as to perform in sports. "The pressure to start using [steroids] is in high school," says Dr. Linn Goldberg, who has led studies on performance-enhancing drugs for the Oregon Health & Science University in Portland. "You get the influence of older teens in high school, so when you're a 14-year-old that comes in, you have

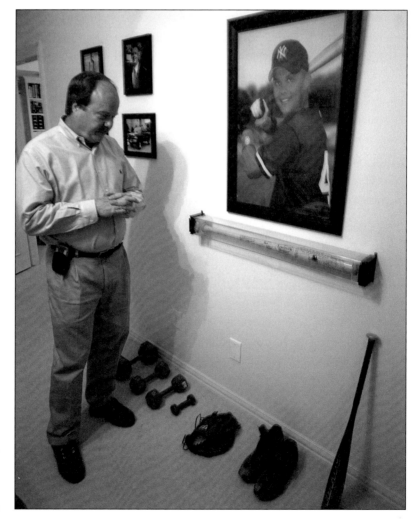

Don Hooton believes the suicide of his seventeen-year-old son Taylor (in photograph) was related to steroid use. Hooton, at one time a fervent advocate of drug testing of student athletes, now urges increased efforts to educate young athletes about the dangers of steroid use.

17-year-olds who are the seniors, and they can have great influence as you progress into the next stage of your athletic career."[52]

In response to this threat, the New Jersey State Interscholastic Athletic Association in 2005 became the first high school association in the country to implement a statewide program of athlete drug testing. Texas and Illinois also test athletes on a statewide basis, and several other states have considered joining suit. Florida implemented drug testing in 2007, but the program was dropped after only one year due to budget constraints. Similarly, when the program in Texas began in the 2007–2008 school year, it was the largest high school drug program in the country, but it has since shrunk to about a third of its original size. In a survey of schools undertaken by the National Federation of State High School Associations (NFHS), more than half of the schools said that they did not have a drug-testing program because they lacked financial resources.

These examples demonstrate that one of the biggest challenges for high school drug-testing programs is the expense. The New Jersey State Interscholastic Athletic Association spends roughly $100,000 per year to test roughly five hundred student athletes during state championship events. The rate of positive tests has never exceeded 1 percent. During the first year of the high school drug-testing program in Illinois (2008–2009), the Illinois High School Association spent $100,000 to test 650 students. Illinois had not a single positive result that first year.

In most other states, testing is left up to individual school districts. It is impossible to know how many districts have drug-testing policies in place, but experts agree that the number is growing. A 2008 survey undertaken by NFHS revealed that over 13 percent of high schools had a policy in place for drug testing, and another 17 percent had programs in the planning phases. Roughly two-thirds of these programs focused only on student athletes.

It is difficult to justify spending tax money on this expense, particularly when the rate of drug detection is so low. In fact, several school districts have ended their student drug-testing programs due to the expense. Dublin County, Ohio, for instance, ended its drug testing program and reallocated the $35,000 it was spending per year to hire two new substance abuse counselors.

"As the father of a middle-school student athlete, I firmly believe participation in sports is, in and of itself, a deterrent to drug use," writes one blogger. "[S]tudent athletes are the least likely among their peers to be using drugs and alcohol."[53]

Comprehensive Testing

Drug Free Sport is the biggest provider of drug testing for colleges and high schools. The most comprehensive menu of drugs that Drug Free Sport tests for costs about $150 per test; a less expensive option ($80) tests for about twenty substances. Neither of these tests includes peptide hormones (nonsteroid hormones that are the building blocks for protein), stimulants, narcotics, or masking agents. "Are we missing some kids because we're not doing the full WADA list? Absolutely," admits Wickerham. "But if you're going to do a drug test, it's better to do some drug testing than none."[54] In fact, some schools use tests more commonly associated with employer screening programs than athlete drug tests. These generally focus on illegal drugs. The cost of a standard Substance Abuse Panel (SAP-10) that screens for ten common drugs ranges from $25 to $50 per test.

Rather than include more agents to be tested for in each test, schools have generally preferred to invest in programs with a broader reach. Most schools with drug-testing programs begin with the sports with the highest likelihood of drug use and expand outward to other sports and related clubs such as cheerleading or spirit teams. A number of schools have broadened drug-testing programs beyond athletes to test students participating in other extracurricular activities—everything from music programs to drama to chess club. The Supreme Court has struck down laws that would force a student who has been suspended from school to submit to a drug test because it violates that student's right to an education, but extracurricular activities are beyond the scope of this constitutional right. In *Board of Education v. Earls* (2002), the Supreme Court upheld the right of schools to require students involved in any extracurricular activities to participate in drug tests.

"Are we missing some kids because we're not doing the full WADA list? Absolutely. But if you're going to do a drug test, it's better to do some drug testing than none."[54]

— Andrea Wickerham, the vice president of Drug Free Sport.

Statewide High School Drug-Testing Programs

Three states currently have drug-testing programs for high school athletes. In 2006 New Jersey became the first state to establish a program. New Jersey's program applies only to athletes who belong to teams that qualify for statewide tournaments. Athletes who test positive are banned from competition for one year. Illinois's program, which was established by the Illinois High School Association, began in 2008. The program conducts random testing of athletes competing in sectional, regional, and championship games.

The program in Texas was established by an act of the state legislature and is the most far-reaching of the state programs. It covers more than forty thousand athletes in all sports and includes random testing of 3 percent of these athletes. Texas uses a tiered approach to penalties. The first positive result receives a thirty-day suspension, the second a one-year suspension. If an athlete tests positive three times, he or she is permanently banned from competition.

Some advocates of athlete drug testing believe that the tests should continue to focus exclusively on performance-enhancing substances. The state court of California ruled that testing should be allowed for student athletes who expected their physical condition to be scrutinized, but that testing students in academic clubs, band, or other extracurricular activities violates the privacy protections in the state's constitution.

How Parents Feel About Drug Testing

The testing policies at high schools and middle schools are somewhat different than those for elite athletes. Testing protocol allows students privacy as they provide a urine sample. But some parents believe the requirement is a violation of a student's rights to privacy just the same. When a seventh grader at Delaware Valley Middle School in Millford, Pennsylvania, brought home a permission slip for a drug test as part of her application to participate in an afterschool program, her mom was outraged. "They were asking a 12-year-old to pee in a cup," says mom Kathy Kiederer. "I have a problem with that. They're violating her right to privacy."[55]

Administrators say that parents who disapprove are in the minority, however. Prior to implementing its drug-testing program for middle and high school students in 2011, the Maryville School District in Missouri surveyed parents, and more than 72 percent of respondents said that a drug-testing program was necessary.

Linn State Technical College, a two-year public college in Missouri, took drug testing to another level when it adopted a policy in 2011 to require all incoming students to take a drug test. Students were required to pay fifty dollars to cover the cost of the test, and those who refused to take the test were threatened with administrative withdrawal from the college. The measure met with considerable opposition from parents, students, and the American Civil Liberties Union (ACLU), which filed a lawsuit on the students' behalf. At preliminary hearings, the judge ordered the college to halt the drug tests, but the case is making its way through the appeals system.

When Student Athletes Test Positive

Athlete drug testing at all levels usually includes illegal street drugs like marijuana, cocaine, and opiates as well as substances more often associated with performance enhancement. Testing for illegal drugs is not limited to student athletes; they are on the list of banned substances used by WADA, the IOC, and most professional sports organizations as well. The difference is that street drugs are more likely to be the main target of athlete drug programs at the high school and college levels than they are at the Olympics or in professional sports. This is reflected in the sanctions. According to NCAA rules, athletes who test positive for drugs lose one year of eligibility for their first offense and are withheld from competition for a full season. A second positive test for a performance-enhancing drug results in a total ban from competition; a second positive test for a street drug results in the loss of a second year of competition. The difference in the sanctions for use of performance-enhancing versus street drugs demonstrates the

Challenges to School-Based Drug-Testing Policies

The American Civil Liberties Union is among the organizations that have challenged the right of schools to conduct mandatory drug tests for students. Lawyers argue that mandatory testing is a violation of a student's right to privacy. They further argue that drug testing is constitutional only when there is a reason for suspicion. Some people say that "suspicionless" drug testing of high school students engaged in extracurricular activities is aimed at the students least likely to get in trouble with drugs and will scare away youth at risk for drug use from participating in after-school programs, which have been proved to be effective drug-prevention tools.

The Supreme Court has ruled on this issue several times. In the 1995 case *Vernonia School District 47J v. Acton*, the court upheld the policy of an Oregon school to conduct drug testing of student athletes. In a 2002 case the court overruled an appeals court that had decided that the Tecumseh, Oklahoma, Public School District's drug-testing policy was unconstitutional. The policy required high school students participating in any extracurricular activities—academic, artistic, and so on—to submit to drug tests. The federal court had ruled this policy to be unconstitutional because there was no suspicion that any of the students tested had ever used illegal drugs or that the school had a widespread drug problem.

dual goals of drug testing at the collegiate level. Eliminating an athlete who is using performance-enhancing drugs is considered integral to ensuring fairness within the sport; greater leniency with regard to street drugs suggests that the goal of testing for these is to identify drug use for intervention.

Within individual schools, approaches for dealing with a positive test result vary. Almost all schools inform the parents of a student the first time that he or she tests positive for drugs. Most schools refer students to a substance abuse course, drug counseling, or similar intervention program. Some may also include community service or similar punishment. At the University of Oregon, for instance, student athletes who test positive are required to participate in a counseling and education program; a second positive test results in a "behavior modification contract" between the student and the coach. Student athletes who test positive for drugs often become the target for subsequent tests, perhaps on a monthly basis. Students may be required to pay for the costs that are incurred as part of these sanctions.

Most athlete drug tests look for illegal street drugs as well as performance-enhancing drugs. The goal of testing college-level athletes for illegal street drugs such as marijuana is intervention. The goal of testing these athletes for performance-enhancing drugs is keeping competition fair.

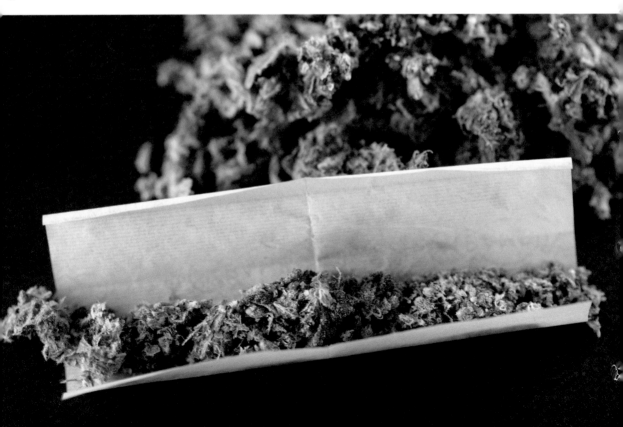

Expulsion or suspension from sports and/or other extracurricular activities is common. In a recent survey conducted by the NFHS, roughly 85 percent of high schools reported that a positive drug test resulted in mandatory suspension from competition or dismissal from an activity.

At the high school level, parents are sometimes integral to the solution. At South Beloit School District #320 in Illinois, for example, the first time a student athlete tests positive for drugs the parents are informed, the student is suspended from sports for eight weeks, and both parents and the student are required to participate in counseling. After the eight-week suspension the student is eligible to resume activities but is targeted for future drug testing. If a student athlete self-reports a problem with drug use, the student can retain his or her eligibility as long as the student and parents attend the eight-week counseling sessions.

By law, results of a positive drug test are confidential. Law enforcement is not involved unless students are selling or distributing the drugs. In adherence with the Family Educational Rights and Privacy Act, the drug test results are expunged when the student graduates from or leaves high school.

Some antidrug advocates worry that drug-testing programs may undermine the very goal that they set out to achieve. Some students may be embarrassed, wary, or otherwise uncomfortable about providing a sample and decide joining the team or participating in the activity is not worth the discomfort. By dissuading students from participating in after-school activities, the tests may push these students away from positive, organized, self-esteem-building activities, increasing the likelihood that they will become more socially isolated, one of the risk factors for illegal drug use. "If we only drug test students in athletics and extracurricular activities, and they might be experimenting or smoking a little pot, we're actually driving them away from participating in those activities," argues Kris Krane, the executive director of Students for Sensible Drug Policy. "I think these kinds of policies actually create more drug abuse among young people."[56]

> "If we only drug test students in athletics and extracurricular activities, and they might be experimenting or smoking a little pot, we're actually driving them away from participating in those activities."[56]
>
> — Kris Krane, executive director of Students for Sensible Drug Policy.

Drug Tests as a Deterrent for Student Athletes

The main reason that most high schools and middle schools employ drug testing is not to catch athletes who are cheating but rather to stop students from doing drugs in the first place. Jerry Cecil, the superintendent of the Greenwood School District in Arkansas, which has an aggressive testing program for student athletes, says, "We don't want to catch students. We want them not to be using."[57]

Experts have widely different opinions about whether drug tests serve as a deterrent. Some say that the possibility of being tested positive for drugs dissuades young people from using them and offers students a way to say no to drugs. As evidence they point to the low rate of positive tests. (The rate of positive tests in NCAA's drug-testing program has never been higher than 1 percent in any year.) Matthew Franz, who owns Sport Safe, a drug-testing company in Columbus, Ohio, warns that drug use "starts early with kids. You want to get in there and plant these seeds of what's out there and do prevention early. The 11th and 12th graders, most of them have already made a choice. But the eighth graders, they're still making decisions, and it helps if you give them that deterrent."[58]

At the core of this controversy is whether the thousands of dollars spent each year on drug testing has any advantage. Take the program in Illinois, for example. The Illinois High School Association, which began its drug-testing program in the 2008–2009 school year, spends about $100,000 annually to test roughly 650 students. As of late 2012 the program has never had a positive result. Executive Director Kurt Gibson sees this as a positive: "We continue to view that our program is accomplishing what it set out to do," he says. "It's another tool in the student's toolbox to say no to these substances. Our program serves more as a deterrent rather than being designed to punish students."[59]

Some experts say such thinking is illogical. "If you're using drug testing to weed out a problem in kids, you need to get them in therapy. But it doesn't reduce whether or not kids use drugs,"

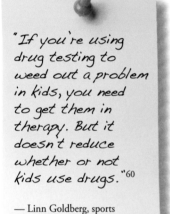

"If you're using drug testing to weed out a problem in kids, you need to get them in therapy. But it doesn't reduce whether or not kids use drugs."[60]

— Linn Goldberg, sports medicine expert.

concludes Linn Goldberg. "Drug testing has never been shown to have a deterrent effect."[60]

Some drug-prevention experts argue that drug testing may also undermine the effectiveness of antidrug efforts and treatment programs. "School drug testing really breaks down the trust between students and teachers, counselors, and administrators," says a student who has lobbied for alternatives to drug testing. "If [students] do have a substance abuse problem, they need to see authority figures as people they can trust, not as people constantly viewing them as suspects. Drug testing tells these kids they're guilty until proven innocent."[61]

Although experts disagree about how to rid schools and sports of drugs, most experts agree that it is far easier to stop drug use before it starts. Thus, testing at the high school level and catching athletes using performance-enhancing drugs may be an integral part of a larger drug prevention strategy that includes education and information.

Facts

- The NCAA spends roughly $4.5 million a year to collect and analyze approximately 13,500 samples through its drug-testing program, and an additional $1.5 million on drug education programs.

- Respondents to a 2009 poll of colleges and universities reported that the majority of drug-testing samples taken from students are tested for marijuana (95 percent), cocaine and amphetamines (94 percent), narcotics (83 percent), ecstasy (74 percent), ephedrine (67 percent), and anabolic agents (22 percent).

- The NCAA tests at championship events in all three divisions at least once every five years, and some championships are tested every year. At these events about twenty-five hundred student athletes are screened annually for steroids, diuretics and masking agents, stimulants, and other performance-enhancing drugs. Street drugs such as marijuana and cocaine are also typically included in the drug tests.

- Today 90 percent of Division I, 65 percent of Division II, and 21 percent of Division III schools conduct their own drug-testing program in addition to the NCAA's.

- Studies show that the number of high schools implementing new drug-testing programs is escalating; today, between 20 and 27 percent of high schools have some type of drug-testing program in place.

- In a 2008 survey undertaken by the NFHS, 54 percent of schools said they did not have a drug-testing program because they lacked financial resources, and 51 percent said they lacked school board approval.

- In an NCAA survey of colleges, 69 percent of respondents have a treatment plan in place for student athletes who test positive for drug use; another 7 percent were actively creating such a plan.

- In a survey conducted by NFHS, 98 percent of schools said they inform parents of a student's positive drug test, and 92 percent of schools with drug-testing programs refer students testing positive for drug use to counseling or rehabilitation programs.

Is Drug Testing Effective in Reducing Drug Use Among Athletes?

The primary goal of drug testing for young people and elite athletes alike is to put a stop to the use of drugs. Sanctions and punishments for a positive test are designed toward this end, but experts disagree about whether the consequences of one, two, or even more positive tests are sufficient to stop athletes from using performance-enhancing substances.

Getting Away With It

Part of the problem is that most athletes do not expect to get caught. At the high school and college levels, far more athletes are not selected for tests than are, even during the championship events. And even though Olympic athletes know they will be subjected to rigorous testing protocols, the number who are caught cheating suggests that many assume their number will not come up—or hope for the best in case it does. During the six months prior to the 2012 London Olympics, 117 athletes received sanctions for drug offenses, and nine additional positive drug tests occurred during the Games themselves.

Athletes also may believe that they will be able to beat the tests. At the most elite levels of sport, such thinking is sometimes backed up by coaches, doctors, and colleagues who have sophisticated knowledge that can help them accomplish this task. Experts also say that the drug labs are often one step ahead of the tests, so that top athletes may have in their arsenal designer drugs for which there is no test.

Some experts say that rather than deterring the use of existing drugs, the drug tests encourage athletes to find new substances that are not subject to testing. "The use of THG (tetrahydrogestrinone or 'the clear'), is an anabolic steroid created in a laboratory, designed to avoid detection," says Linn Goldberg in expert testimony to Congress. "Use was successfully masked until a sample of THG was sent to the Olympic laboratory for analysis and a number of athletes were identified as steroid users when their urine samples were reexamined. For those athletes, drug testing did not deter use, but resulted in searching for methods to beat the test."[62] Similarly, recent evidence suggests that drug use was rampant among cyclists in the Tour de France, but that more aggressive drug testing caused more secretive and more systemized drug use among some teams.

> "If people want to continue to do what they shouldn't do, then the one thing that you have to do is you have to have stricter penalties. It's as simple as that."[64]
>
> — Bud Selig, commissioner of Major League Baseball.

Many people say that the drug tests are too few and far between for them to provide any real deterrent for athletes intent on cheating. "While they know that using drugs is illegal, athletes will not stop unless there are consequences or a significant possibility of getting caught," writes one teen athlete. "[Drug use] is against the rules and should be dealt with harshly . . . a zero-tolerance policy should be in place at all levels of competition."[63]

Some experts agree with this teen that one of the reasons drug use persists is that the consequences of testing positive for drug use are insufficient deterrents. Bud Selig, the commissioner of MLB, says that harsh penalties are the only way to keep people from cheating. "If people want to continue to do what they shouldn't

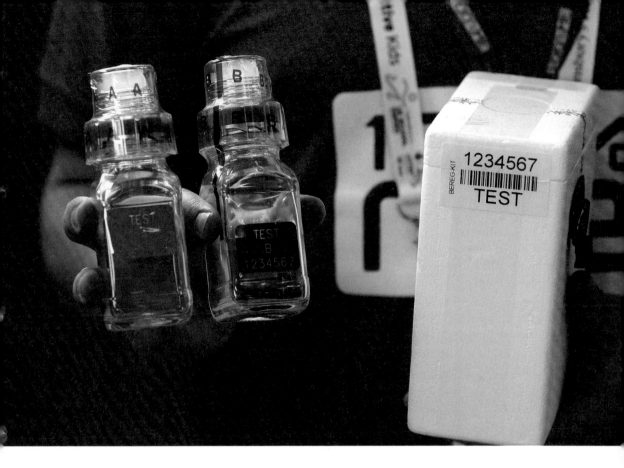

do, then the one thing that you have to do is you have to have stricter penalties," he told reporters in a 2013 press conference. "It's as simple as that."[64]

The Impact on an Athlete's Reputation

Ideally, the notion of being labeled as a cheater would deter the use of banned substances among elite athletes. To this end, sports-governing entities at the Olympic and professional levels usually publicize the names of athletes who test positive for banned substances. Some sports organizations also release the name of the substance for which the athlete tested positive, although collective bargaining agreements sometimes prohibit this. The assumption is that the negative publicity that results from a positive drug test may serve as a deterrent.

Yet although getting caught using drugs can bring athletes the disdain of the public, fans have consistently shown a willingness

Sealed containers holding athlete urine samples await transport to a lab for drug analysis. Even athletes who know they will be subjected to rigorous testing sometimes flout the rules and hope for the best.

Drug Testing and Boxing

Unlike most other professional sports in the United States, boxing has no governing authority or Olympic committee in charge of drug testing. The sport is governed by boxing commissions in each state, which generally consider themselves to be outside WADA jurisdiction. Boxing has been plagued with allegations of widespread anabolic steroid use as well as use of human growth hormones, tetrahydrogestrinone (THG), and diuretics that may help boxers move to a lower weight division.

For many years the only drug testing for boxers has consisted of tests immediately before and after a fight. The problem with this system is that these athletes have medical advisers who know how to taper off the use of steroids and other drugs. Many lovers of the sport, including match organizers and boxers themselves, say it is time for stricter drug-testing procedures that would include random drug testing. In response, the Nevada State Athletic Commission has begun to implement random drug testing, but athletes are given advance notice—a step that experts say minimizes its effectiveness. Given the high payoffs and the danger of the sport, it may only be a matter of time before boxing joins other professional sports in implementing random drug testing for athletes at all levels.

to forgive the athletes they love for their transgressions. Amid suspicions of drug use by Sammy Sosa and Mark McGwire during their 1998 chase for the home run record, many people said they did not care whether the extra power the athletes were getting was due to steroids—it was fun to watch. Later admissions of drug use did little to change popular opinion, and many fans believe the great hitters should be admitted into the Hall of Fame regardless of whether their success was fueled by drug use.

A related issue deals with the rewards for athletes. Athletes compete to win. They want the coveted gold medal or brass ring. They want to see their names etched in the history books, not as a cheater but as a winner. Some drug-testing advocates believe that prohibiting this from happening—stripping athletes of their medals or barring them from the hall of fame—will also serve as a deterrent. Thus, at the Olympic level, a positive test results in an athlete's being stripped of a medal—usually immediately but sometimes many years later—medals for which most Olympic athletes have worked all their lives.

The issue of whether record-busting baseball players suspected of steroid use should be allowed in the Hall of Fame has not been decided. Given MLB's efforts to clean up the sport's image future sanctions for positive drug tests will likely include being banned from baseball's Hall of Fame. In January 2013, Hall of Fame candidates Barry Bonds and Roger Clemens fell far short of the votes needed to be inducted, receiving just 36.2 percent and 37.6 percent, of "yes" votes, respectively. (To be inducted in the Hall of Fame requires 75 percent of eligible voters to agree.) The reason was not their performance on the field: Bonds held the record for career home runs and pitcher Clemens had a record seven Cy Young Awards (which are given to the year's best pitcher). Though neither man has admitted to steroid use, most analysts agreed that suspicions of steroid use are what kept them out of the Baseball Hall of Fame. "When I vote for a player I am upholding him for the highest individual honor possible," wrote *Sports Illustrated* writer Tom Verducci. "My vote is an endorsement of a career, not part of it, and how it was achieved. Voting for a known steroid user is endorsing steroid use." [65]

The Monetary Impact

Most sports organizations suspend athletes who have tested positive for drug use. Usually, the sanctions become stricter for repeated positive tests, with repeated positive tests resulting in a lifelong suspension. The sanctions are intended to deter drug use among professional athletes in several ways. First, athletes who do not compete are not paid, so a suspension can cost a player hundreds of thousands, or even millions, of dollars. MLB player Carlos Ruiz was suspended for twenty-five games after a second positive test for Adderall, costing him an estimated $750,000 in salary. Manny Ramirez was suspended for fifty games after failing a drug test in May 2009, costing him an estimated $7.7 million in salary.

Beyond the salary loss, being linked to drug use can cost a player lucrative sponsorships and endorsement deals. Olympic swimmer Michael Phelps's public dalliance with marijuana in 2009 cost him several sponsors, most notably Kellogg's. US sprinter Justin Gatlin, who won the 100-meter gold medal in the 2004 Olympics and stood to earn an estimated $2 million to $4 million in annual endorsements and sponsorships, was dropped by his sponsor just three weeks after testing positive for a banned substance in 2006. US cyclist Floyd Landis, who won the 2006 Tour de France, lost the title after testing positive for a performance-enhancing steroid during the competition. In addition, the positive drug test cost him his $3 million contract with sponsor Phonak, $2 million in lost endorsements, and nearly $4 million in prospective endorsements of equipment and lifestyle products as the reigning Tour de France victor.

Teamwork

Just as sponsors may question whether they want to be associated with an athlete who is suspected of drug use, so may prospective teams. A suspension due to a positive drug test, particularly involving a star player who will miss important games, puts a team at a disadvantage. Advocates of drug testing say that this helps to put pressure on teams—the coaches, trainers, doctors, and other players—to ferret out drug use before the player is caught.

Yet, to date, the loss of income and sponsorships appears not to have deterred some athletes from using drugs. If professional athletes have a lot to lose if they are caught using drugs, they may have even more to gain by taking the risk. The same athletes who lose contracts and endorsements worth millions of dollars often believe that the drugs are what got them these opportunities in the first place. Lance Armstrong reportedly earned $12 million from the US Postal Service, his team's sponsor, as the winner of just

Changing Attitudes as a Deterrent

Even among those who believe drug tests to be a deterrent, many say that drug tests alone will be insufficient to control doping. The drug tests need to be accompanied by a profound change in the attitudes of athletes. Not surprisingly, studies have shown that athletes who regard doping as a minor health risk are at greater risk of using drugs than those who say it has significant health risks. Experts have used this information to suggest that a stronger drug-prevention and education program should accompany drug testing.

On the other hand, some studies suggest that the risk a performance-enhancing drug poses may also not be a sufficient deterrent. In 1967, when researcher Gabe Mirkin asked competitive runners whether they would take a drug that would make them an Olympic champion, even if it would kill them within a year, more than half replied that they would take the pill. Although the question posed a hypothetical situation, the continued use of substances that have proved to be dangerous—and even resulted in the death of young, otherwise healthy athletes—suggests that the dilemma is very real.

three of his Tour de France races. Mark McGwire has a net worth upward of $60 million, earned in large part by steroid-fueled hitting. For top-earning athletes fines and suspensions may amount to just a fraction of their life earnings.

Even repeated positive drug tests do not always mean the end of a career. Many athletes are caught using drugs again and again before finally being banned from the sport. Moreover, critics of the current system say that some professional sports organizations may look the other way. In fact, there may not be a real incentive for professional organizers to crack down on drug use or use the tests to catch cheaters. A suspension resulting from a positive drug test is not only bad for athletes and their teams, it can be bad for the sport as well. The suspension of a star player may mean fewer ticket sales, which costs a team money. Ultimately, a sport has at risk the loss of its reputation.

At the college level, student athletes are warned about the dangers of drugs. They are told that drug use could put an end to a promising career. Indeed, they are shown examples where this has happened, such as the tragic 1986 death of promising basketball star Len Bias at the age of twenty-two. Yet, college athletes see a very different situation than this. Again and again, players who have tested positive for drug use are drafted by professional teams anyway. For instance, drug tests are routinely conducted at the football scouting combine, at which professional football teams have an opportunity to look at and interview potential players. A positive test seems to have little or no impact on whether a player is drafted. Six football players tested positive for anabolic steroids at the 2012 scouting combine, for instance, and at least three of them were subsequently drafted by professional teams. Critics say this is both an illustration that drug testing is not working as a deterrent and an explanation of why. "What message does this send to collegiate and high school athletes about toleration of their drug use?"[66] asks Linn Goldberg rhetorically.

What Do the Numbers Mean?

To determine whether drug testing is an effective deterrent to drug use, experts often look at the number of positive results. Proponents of drug testing point to evidence that the use of performance-enhancing drugs appears to be on the wane. An NCAA survey undertaken every four years showed a decline between 2005 and 2009 in the percentage of athletes using anabolic steroids (from 1.1 percent to 0.4 percent) and amphetamines (from 4.2 percent to 3.7 percent). Moreover, the rate of positive drug tests has remained relatively stable over the years.

Others say that drug testing has little or nothing to do with the downward trend in drug use among student athletes. While less than 1 percent of NCAA athletes test positive for drug use, the most recent NCAA survey of student athletes (2009) revealed that 22.6 percent of athletes had used marijuana within the last twelve months—a 1.4 percentage point increase over 2005. In addition, 3.3 percent of respondents indicated that they had used narcotics, and over half of the users took the drugs both during their competitive season and their off-season. With regard to performance-enhancing drugs, 3.7 percent of the respondents indicated that they had used amphetamines, with over half of them indicating that they had used the amphetamines during both their competitive and their off-season, although most had used them after practice and/or competition. In addition, less than one-half of one percent of respondents (0.4 percent) had used anabolic steroids within the last twelve months. The majority of the students who used steroids said they did so during the off-season.

The question is whether more athletes would take performance-enhancing drugs if drug tests were not in place. The answer to this question is almost impossible to know, and experts have come to opposite conclusions. In a study undertaken at Brigham Young University, researchers found that roughly 12 percent of athletes would use steroids under the "right circumstances," which were "largely defined as the ability to achieve their athletic potential without testing positive for use."[67] The authors concluded that "testing itself, although an effective deterrent to drug use, may not eliminate drug use among college athletes. . . . In general, the decision to not use drugs is felt to be related more to the fear of reprisal than to health issues, and users continue to look for ways to avoid detection rather than decide not to use these banned substances."[68]

Some experts point to a decline in positive tests as evidence that fewer athletes are using drugs. Yet, a decline in positive results may not mean that fewer people are taking performance-enhancing drugs but rather that more people are using drugs for which there is not yet a test or have figured out another way to beat the tests. Don Catlin has become disillusioned with drug testing at the college level. "If a guy or girl wants to beat the test, there are perfectly well-known ways of doing that," he says in a 2013 interview. "The

"All these negative tests lead us to the conclusion that there's no drug problem. I would almost rather see no testing at all."[69]

— Don Hooton, father of a seventeen-year-old whose suicide was blamed on steroid use.

athletes know when the tests are going to take place. They get sick or they don't show up. . . . I think the whole drug-testing industry deserves a bad review."[69]

Don Hooton, who blames his son's suicide on anabolic steroids, was once a fervent advocate of drug testing for high school athletes. He has recently questioned whether the drug tests are having the desired effect, however. "All these negative tests lead us to the conclusion that there's no drug problem," says Hooton. "I would almost rather see no testing at all."[70]

What the Research Suggests

Several researchers have been going beyond simple numbers in an effort to determine whether random drug testing is in fact a deterrent to drug use among young people. Again, different studies have come to different conclusions. In 2007 the US Department of Education engaged the Mathematica Policy Research group in Princeton, New Jersey, to explore whether drug testing discouraged

Athletes who have been linked to drug use have lost lucrative sponsorships and endorsements. Olympic swimmer Michael Phelps (shown here during the 2008 Olympics) lost Kellogg's as a sponsor after public dalliance with marijuana.

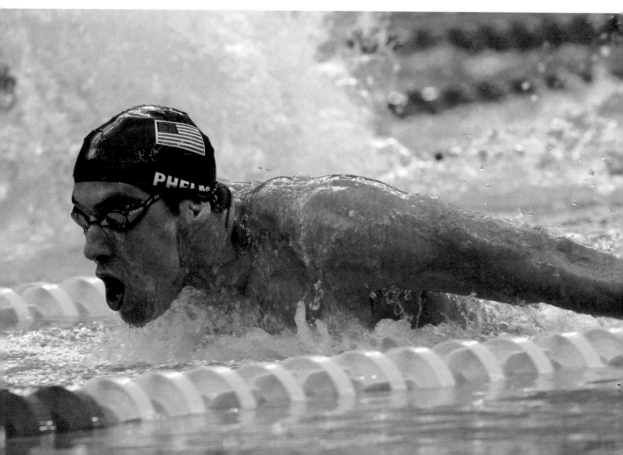

drug use. In this largest empirical evaluation to date, researchers compared eighteen schools that had mandatory random student drug testing to eighteen comparable schools without drug tests.

The findings, published in the February 2012 issue of the *Journal of Adolescent Health*, showed that students subject to the tests reported less substance use compared to the students where there was no drug testing. The authors also report, "We found no evidence of unintentional negative effects on students' future intentions to use substances, the proportion of students who participated in activities subject to drug testing, or on students' attitudes toward school and perceived consequences of substance use."[71] The results were confined to the students who were subject to testing, however; there were no spillover effects for other students.

The findings are in direct contrast to a 2009 research project undertaken by the Oregon Health & Science University. The SATURN (Student Athlete Testing Using Random Notification) study compared drug use among athletes at five high schools that had drug-testing programs with athletes at six schools without a drug-testing program in place. The study found no difference in alcohol or drug consumption in the two groups. "Random drug and alcohol testing does not reliably keep student-athletes from using," said the research team. "In fact, the mere presence of drug testing increases some risk factors for future substance use," researchers said. The SATURN project also found that "athletes at schools with drug and alcohol testing felt less athletically competent, perceived school authorities were less opposed to drug use, and believed less in the benefits of drug testing."[72]

A telephone survey undertaken by researchers at the University of Pennsylvania in 2007 and 2008 concurred that drug tests in high schools had minimal impact on drug and alcohol use among teens. Overall, 27 percent of the students said their schools engaged in drug testing. The survey showed no evidence that drug-testing policies led male students to avoid drugs.

Drug-testing policies seemed to have a minor impact on female

> "Random drug and alcohol testing does not reliably keep student-athletes from using. In fact, the mere presence of drug testing increases some risk factors for future substance use."[71]
>
> — Researchers at the Oregon Health & Science University.

students, but only in schools where rules are clear and enforced and student-adult relationships are based on respect. Female students in schools that test for drugs, but in which students distrust adults and where there are other social problems, may actually use drugs more than those in comparable schools without drug testing. Dan Romer, coauthor of the study, warns:

> This study sends a cautionary note to the estimated 20% or more of high schools that have joined the drug testing bandwagon. We find little evidence that this approach to minimizing teen drug use is having the deterrent effect its proponents claim. And only in schools that have a very good school climate, reported by about a third of students, does this intervention exert a protective influence on adolescent girls. Schools that have joined the rush to implement testing should ask themselves whether this strategy has been oversold.[73]

"We find little evidence that this [drug testing] approach to minimizing teen drug use is having the deterrent effect its proponents claim."[72]

— Dan Romer, researcher at the University of Pennsylvania's Annenberg Public Policy Center.

The Future of Drug Testing

Despite concerns about its effectiveness in deterring drug use among the world's best and the country's youngest athletes, drug testing is no doubt here to stay. History suggests that athletes will continue to find ways to improve their performance, and in doing so a few will decide to break the rules. History also suggests that scientists and policy makers will continue to look for ways to stop the cheaters with new tests and more stringent testing procedures.

While drug testing is a critical tool, public opinion may be even more important. If society decides that performance-enhancing drugs are a natural part of the sport, the bans may gradually be lifted. If, on the other hand, society decides that it is more important to protect the health of athletes, the cat and mouse chase that drug testing has become will continue. The game is on.

Facts

- Experts at the University of Mainz advise that it would take as many as 150 drug tests to catch the average drug user.

- In a 2010 study 7 percent of athletes admitted to using doping substances, but only 0.8 percent had failed random drug tests.

- In a survey of athletes published in the 2010 *International Journal of Drug Policy*, 76 percent of athletes said that drug testing was an effective deterrent to drug use.

- In a 2008 Gallup Poll 50 percent of respondents said the IOC was doing enough to curb drug use among Olympic athletes, but 44 percent said it was not.

- In the 2010–2011 academic year, 10,735 athletes were tested in the NCAA's year-round program. There were sixty-three positive tests, a rate of 0.6 percent.

- In a 2009 survey conducted by the NCAA, 55 percent of student athletes said they agreed or strongly agreed that testing deterred athletes from using drugs.

- In a 2009 survey conducted by the NCAA, 61 percent of respondents strongly agreed or agreed that imposing team penalties for positive drug tests is fair and appropriate.

- In a 2009 survey of college athletes, over 82 percent of respondents indicated that they strongly agreed or agreed that all professional athletes should be tested for drugs, and roughly 89 percent strongly agreed or agreed that all Olympic athletes should be tested for drug use.

Source Notes

Introduction: A Universal Dilemma

1. Oprah Winfrey Network, "Oprah and Lance Armstrong: The Worldwide Exclusive." www.oprah.com.
2. USADA, "Statement from USADA CEO Travis T. Tygart Regarding the U.S. Postal Service Pro Cycling Team Doping Conspiracy," October 10, 2012. http://cyclinginvestigation.usada.org.
3. Quoted in Tom Goldman, "Lance Armstrong and the Business of Doping," NPR, November 21, 2012. www.npr.org.
4. Quoted in John Hoberman, "Dopers on Wheels: The Tour's Sorry History," MSNBC, September 20, 2007. http://nbcsports.msnbc.com.
5. Quoted in Piers Edwards, "The Gain Game: Why Do Sports Stars Cheat?," CNN.com, December 11, 2012. http://edition.cnn.com.
6. Quoted in Hoberman, "Dopers on Wheels."
7. Robert A. Stinchcomb, "Drug Testing in the World of Interscholastic Athletics," *Coach and Athletic Director*, October 1, 2008. www.thefreelibrary.com.
8. Christie Aschwanden, "The Top Athletes Looking for an Edge and the Scientists Trying to Stop Them," *Smithsonian*, July/August 2012. www.smithsonianmag.com.
9. George Mavrotas, "Anti-Doping from an Athlete's Perspective," WADA Educational Symposium, 2006. www.wada-ama.org.
10. Quoted in WADA, "Athlete Testimonies on Whereabouts System," WADA, March 17, 2009. www.wada-ama.org.

Chapter One: What Are the Origins of the Athlete Drug-Testing Controversy?

11. Quoted in Matt Slater, "Gene Doping: Sport's Next Big Challenge," BBC Sports, June 12, 2008. http://gmathletes.wordpress.com.
12. WADA, "A Brief History of Anti-Doping," June 2010. www.wada-ama.org.
13. Quoted in Christine Brennan, "Babashoff Had Mettle to Speak Out About Steroids," *USA Today*, July 15, 2004. www.usatoday.com.
14. David A. Baron, David M. Martin, and Samir Abol Magd, "Doping in Sports and Its Spread to At-Risk Populations: An International Review," *World Psychiatry*, June 2007. www.ncbi.nlm.nih.gov.

15. Quoted in Juliet Macur and Michael S. Schmidt, "Former Met Is First Player to Test Positive for H.G.H.," *New York Times,* August 18, 2011. http://www.nytimes.com.

16. Quoted in Macur and Schmidt, "Former Met Is First Player to Test Positive for H.G.H."

17. Chris Cooper, *Run, Swim, Throw, Cheat: The Science Behind Drugs in Sport.* Oxford University Press, 2012, p. 103.

18. WADA, "Gene Doping," October 2009. www.wada-ama.org.

19. Quoted in Helen Branswell, "Experts Warn Gene Doping in Sport 'Inevitable' as Science Advances," MSN, February 4, 2010. http://news.ca.msn .com.

20. WADA, "Gene Doping," October 2009. www.wada-ama.org.

21. John Fahey, "President's Welcome Message," World Anti-Doping Agency, August 2010. www.wada-ama.org.

Chapter Two: How Big a Problem Is Drug Use in Sports?

22. John William Devine, "Doping Is a Threat to Sporting Excellence," *British Journal of Sports Medicine*, vol. 45, 2011, p. 637. http://bjsm.bmj.com.

23. Quoted in WADA, "Athlete Testimonies on Whereabouts System."

24. Quoted in Ian Steadman, "Why Sports Would Be Better with Doping," *Wired*, September 10, 2012. www.wired.com.

25. Quoted in WADA, "Athlete Testimonies on Whereabouts System."

26. Quoted in Steadman, "Why Sports Would Be Better with Doping."

27. Julian Savulescu, Bennett Foddy, and M. Clayton, "Why We Should Allow Performance Enhancing Drugs in Sport," *British Journal of Sports Medicine*, 2004, p. 38. http://bjsm.bmj.com.

28. Quoted in Peter Handrinos, "Baseball Men: The Skeptic," Scout.com, December 18, 2006. http://stlcardinals.scout.com.

29. Secrétariat au Loisir et au Sport, "Doping! There's Nothing Sporting About It." www.mels.gouv.qc.ca.

30. Thomas H. Murray, "Sports Enhancement," Hastings Center, 2010. www.thehastingscenter.org.

31. Linn Goldberg, testimony before the U.S. House of Representatives Committee on Oversight and Governmental Reform, "HGH Testing in the NFL," December 12, 2012. http://oversight.house.gov.

32. Stinchcomb, "Drug Testing in the World of Interscholastic Athletics."

33. Nora D. Volkow, "Anabolic Steroid Abuse," National Institute on Drug Abuse, August 2006. www.drugabuse.gov.

34. Taylor Hooton Foundation, "There Are No Shortcuts to Success!," http:// taylorhooton.org.

Chapter Three: How Fair and Reliable Are Drug-Testing Methods and Policies?

35. Caroline Hatton, e-mail to ProCon.org, in "Sports and Drugs: 192 Banned Performance Enhancing Substances and Methods, with Pros & Cons of their Health Effects," ProCon.org, March 12, 2010.

36. MBannon, "USADA and Drug Tests," post, Slowtwitch.com, January 12, 2010. http://forum.slowtwitch.com.

37. Jonathan Mahler, "Lance Armstrong's Confession Is Just the Start," *Bloomberg View,* January 16, 2013. www.bloomberg.com.

38. Quoted in "Jones Pleads Guilty, Admits Lying About Steroids," NBC Sports, October 5, 2007, p. 2. http://nbcsports.msnbc.com.

39. Mavrotas, "Anti-Doping from an Athlete's Perspective."

40. Quoted in Philip Wolf, "Fighting Drug Use by Elite Athletes Is Simply a Losing Battle," *Ottawa Citizen,* February 10, 2010. www.ottawacitizen. com.

41. Quoted in Nick Zaccardi, "An In-Depth Look at the Intricacies of Olympic Drug Testing," *SI.com,* August 23, 2011. http://sportsillustrated.cnn. com.

42. Quoted in Zaccardi, "An In-Depth Look at the Intricacies of Olympic Drug Testing."

43. Quoted in Zaccardi, "An In-Depth Look at the Intricacies of Olympic Drug Testing."

44. Quoted in WADA, "Athlete Testimonies on Whereabouts System."

45. Quoted in Ken Belson and Michael S. Schmidt, "Star Player First to Win Appeal on a Drug Test," *New York Times,* February 24, 2012, p. A1.

46. Quoted in ESPN.com, "Ryan Braun Wins Appeal of Suspension," February 24, 2012. http://espn.go.com.

47. Travis T. Tygart, in Chris Doorley, "Inside a Sports Drug Testing Lab," *Inside Nova,* August 14, 2012. www.pbs.org.

48. Quoted in Belson and Schmidt, "Star Player First to Win Appeal on a Drug Test."

49. Quoted in Mary Pilon, "Drug-Testing Company Tied to N.C.A.A. Stirs Criticism," *New York Times,* January 5, 2013. www.nytimes.com.

Chapter Four: What Role Should Drug Testing Play in Student Athletics?

50. Quoted in Mary Pilon, "Drug-Testing Company Tied to N.C.A.A. Stirs Criticism."

51. Brian Hendrickson, "An Inside Look: How Drug Testing Works," NCAA, August 6, 2012. www.ncaa.org.

52. Quoted in "5 Percent of Youth Have Used Steroids to Bulk Up, Study Finds," FoxNews.com, November 19, 2012. www.foxnews.com.

53. Gestault, "Suspicionless Drug Testing of Students," *Daily Kos*, May 6, 2013. www.dailykos.com.

54. Quoted in Pilon, "Drug-Testing Company Tied to N.C.A.A. Stirs Criticism."

55. Quoted in Mary Pilon, "Middle Schools Add a Team Rule: Get a Drug Test," *New York Times*, September 22, 2012. www.nytimes.com.

56. Quoted in Phillip Smith, "Feature: Number of Schools Embracing Random Drug Testing on the Rise—So Is Opposition," StoptheDrugWar.org, September 26, 2008. http://stopthedrugwar.org.

57. Quoted in Pilon, "Middle Schools Add a Team Rule: Get a Drug Test."

58. Quoted in Pilon, "Middle Schools Add a Team Rule: Get a Drug Test."

59. Quoted in Pilon, "Differing Views on Value of High School Tests."

60. Quoted in Pilon, "Middle Schools Add a Team Rule: Get a Drug Test."

61. Quoted in Smith, "Feature: Number of Schools Embracing Random Drug Testing on the Rise—So Is Opposition."

Chapter Five: Is Drug Testing Effective in Reducing Drug Use Among Athletes?

62. Goldberg, testimony.

63. Taylor M. Wyckoff, "Drug Testing," *Teen Ink*. http://teenink.com.

64. Quoted in "Major League Baseball Chief Wants Stricter Drug Penalties," *Chicago Tribune*, March 3, 2013. www.chicagotribune.com.

65. Quoted in Tyler Kepner, "Bonds (and Everyone) Strikes Out," *New York Times,* January 9, 2013. http://nytimes.com.

66. Goldberg, testimony.

67. Russell Meldrum and Judy R. Feinberg, "Drug Use by College Athletes: Is Random Testing an Effective Deterrent?," *Sport Journal*, United States Sports Academy.

68. Meldrum and Feinberg, "Drug Use by College Athletes."

69. Quoted in Pilon, "Drug-Testing Company Tied to N.C.A.A. Stirs Criticism."

70. Quoted in Pilon, "Differing Views on Value of High School Tests."

71. Susanne James-Burdumy, Brian Goesling, John Deke, and Eric Einspruch, "The Effectiveness of Mandatory-Random Student Drug Testing: A Cluster Randomized Trial," *Journal of Adolescent Health*, vol. 50, no. 2, February 2012, pp. 172–78.

72. Oregon Health & Science University, "Random Drug Testing Not Reliable in Keeping Teen Athletes from Using," February 21, 2011. www.ohsu.edu.

73. Quoted in The Annenberg Public Policy Center of the University of Pennsylvania, "Student Drug Testing Only Shows Effects Among Girls in High Schools with Good Social Climates; Regardless of Climate, No Deterrent Effect for Boys, National Study Finds," press release, August 17, 2011. www.annenbergpublicpolicycenter.org.

Related Organizations and Websites

Association Against Steroid Abuse

521 N. Sam Houston Pkwy. E., Suite 635
Houston, TX 77060
phone: (291) 999-9934
website: www.steroidabuse.com

The mission of the Association Against Steroid Abuse is to educate and safeguard against the abuse of anabolic steroids by providing information about and statistics on the dangers and issues relating to their use.

Athletes Against Steroids

731 Kirkman Rd.
Orlando, FL 32811
phone: (877) 914-9910
website: www.AthletesAgainstSteroids.org

Athletes Against Steroids is an outreach and educational organization dedicated to eradicating steroids in sports.

Community Anti-Drug Coalitions of America (CADCA)

625 Slaters Ln., Suite 300
Alexandria, VA 22314
phone: (800) 542-2322
fax: (703) 706-0565
website: www.cadca.org

The CADCA was created in 1992 to train local grassroots groups in community problem-solving strategies to address local substance abuse–related problems.

National Center for Drug-Free Sport
2537 Madison Ave.
Kansas City, MO 64108
phone: (816) 474-8655
fax: (816) 502-9287
website: www.drugfreesport.com

This organization provides drug-testing services, screening policies, and education programs. Clients include the National Collegiate Athletic Association, Major League Baseball's minor league program, the Professional Golf Association tour, and hundreds of universities and high school associations and conferences.

National Coalition for the Advancement of Drug-Free Athletics (NCADFA)
PO Box 206
New Milford, NJ 07646
phone: (201) 265-8688
website: www.ncadfa.org

The NCADFA's purpose is to support educational, charitable, and scientific organizations engaged in antidrug education and prevention programs. The coalition also provides safe and effective alternatives to help athletes reach their potential.

National Collegiate Athletic Association (NCAA)
700 W. Washington St.
PO Box 6222
Indianapolis, IN 46206-6222
phone: (317) 917-6222
fax: (317) 917-6888
website: www.ncaa.org

The NCAA drug-testing program was created to protect the health and safety of student athletes by ensuring that no participant has an artificially induced advantage or is pressured to use chemical substances.

Partnership for a Drug-Free America
405 Lexington Ave., Suite 1601
New York, NY 10174
phone: (212) 922-1560
fax: (212) 922-1570
website: www.drugfreeamerica.org

The Partnership for a Drug-Free America provides education and awareness programs to prevent young people from using drugs, including performance-enhancing substances. Partnership materials also include a guide for parents and *Coaches Corner*, a blog about healthy sports for young people.

Test Me, I'm Clean
PO Box 31654
Knoxville, TN 37930
website: www.testmeimclean.org

Founded by Olympic gold medalist Dee Dee Trotter, this non-profit organization intends to educate athletes about the dangers of performance-enhancing drugs, to encourage athletes of all ages to stay clean, and to unite in opposition to dishonest athletes.

U.S. Anti-Doping Agency (USADA)
1330 Quail Lake Loop, Suite 260
Colorado Springs, CO 80906-4651
phone: (719) 785-2000
toll-free: (866) 601-2632
fax: (719) 785-2001
website: www.usada.org

Founded in 2000, the USADA serves as the official antidoping agency for Olympic-related sports in the United States and provides education and resources to deter the use of substances among athletes.

World Anti-Doping Agency (WADA)

Stock Exchange Tower
800 Place Victoria, Suite 1700
PO Box 120
Montreal, Quebec H4Z 1B7
Canada
phone: 1-514-904-9232
fax : 1-514-904-8650
website: www.wada-ama.org.

WADA was established in 1999 as an international independent agency composed of sports organizations and governments worldwide. Its key activities include scientific research, education, the development of drug tests and other antidoping measures, and monitoring of the World Anti-Doping Code, which includes a list of prohibited substances and methods.

Additional Reading

Books

Chris Cooper, *Run, Swim, Throw, Cheat: The Science Behind Drugs in Sport*. Oxford University Press, 2012.

Amitava Dasgupta, *Beating Drug Tests and Defending Positive Results: A Toxicologist's Perspective*. New York: Springer, 2010.

Amitava Dasgupta, *Drugs of Abuse: Testing: A Health Educator's Guide to Understanding*. Sudbury, MA: Jones and Bartlett, 2010.

Paul David, *A Guide to the World Anti-Doping Code: A Fight for the Spirit of Sport*. Cambridge University Press, 2008.

Lauri S. Friedman, *Student Drug Testing*. Farmington Hills, MI: Greenhaven, 2011.

Tyler Hamilton and Daniel Coyle, *The Secret Race: Inside the Hidden World of the Tour de France: Doping, Cover-ups, and Winning at All Costs*. New York: Bantam, 2012.

Glen R. Hanson, Peter J. Venturelli, and Annette E. Fleckenstein, *Drugs and Society*. 11th ed. Burlington, MA: Jones & Bartlett Learning, 2012.

Thomas M. Hunt, *Drug Games: The International Olympic Committee and the Politics of Doping, 1960–2008*. Austin: University of Texas Press, 2011.

Mike McNamee and Verner Møller, eds., *Doping and Anti-Doping Policy in Sport: Ethical, Legal, and Social Perspectives*. New York: Routledge, 2011.

Mario Thevis, *Mass Spectronometry in Sports Drug Testing: Characterization of Prohibited Substances and Doping Control Assays.* Hoboken, NJ: John Wiley & Sons, 2010.

Detlef Thieme and Peter Hemmersbach, *Doping in Sports.* Berlin: Springer-Verlag, 2011.

Andrew Tilin, *The Doper Next Door: My Strange and Scandalous Year on Performance-Enhancing Drugs.* Berkeley, CA: Counterpoint, 2011.

Websites

Anabolic Steroid Abuse (www.steroidabuse.org). This National Institute on Drug Abuse website provides links to information and programs related to anabolic steroids and other performance-enhancing drugs.

The Athlete.org (www.theathlete.org). This website, which provides information on drugs, injuries, and exercises for amateur and professional athletes, includes ample information about drug testing in sports.

"Are Steroids Worth the Risk?," Teens Health (www.kidshealth. org/teen/drug_alcohol/drugs/steroids.html). This website includes a wealth of articles and resources on steroid use by teens.

Drug Story.org (www.drugstory.org). This website includes information about the physical and mental effects of steroids and other performance-enhancing drugs, as well as links to other resources and websites.

Drug Testing News (www.drugtestingnews.com). This website is designed to provide the most comprehensive source for up-to-date information on drug and alcohol testing, including legislation and technology.

National Collegiate Athletic Association, Drug Testing (www.ncaa. org/wps/wcm/connect/public/NCAA/Health+and+Safety/ Drug+Testing/Drug+Testing+Landing+Page). This website provides information about NCAA drug-testing policies and practices, including the drugs that are banned, how tests are conducted, and penalties for failing a drug test.

National Institute on Drug Abuse, NIDA for Teens (http://teens. drugabuse.gov/facts/facts_ster1.asp). This site includes basic steroid information for teens, including definitions, hormone information, and possible side effects on the teen body.

"Sports and Drugs," ProCon.org (http://sportsanddrugs.procon. org). This website provides information about the use of drugs among athletes, issues related to whether drug use should be allowed in competition, and expert opinions on both sides of the issue.

Steroid (www.steroid.com). Primarily pro–steroid use, the website provides information on steroids and steroid alternatives, including profiles of various steroids, common side effects, laws related to steroids, history of steroid use, and the use of steroids today in baseball and other sports.

Internet Sources

International Olympic Committee, "Factsheet: The Fight Against Doping and Promotion of Athletes' Health," January 2010. http://sportsanddrugs.procon.org/sourcefiles/IOCFact sheet2010.pdf.

National Institute on Drug Abuse, "Anabolic Steroid Abuse," Research Report Series. www.nida.nih.gov/ResearchReports/ Steroids/AnabolicSteroids.html.

World Anti-Doping Agency, *The World Anti-Doping Code: The 2013 Prohibited List, International Standard*. www.wada-ama .org/Documents/World_Anti-Doping_Program/WADP -Prohibited-list/2013/WADA-Prohibited-List-2013-EN.pdf.

Index

history of use of, in sports, 12–13
prevalence of use of, among
NCAA athletes, 74–75
teens and, 35–37
See also specific drugs
Phelps, Michael, 72, **76**
polls. *See* surveys
Pound, Richard, 29, 32

Raducan, Andrea, 44
Ramirez, Manny, 27
Repoxygen, 22
Romer, Dan, 78
Ruiz, Carlos, 27, 72
Run, Swim, Throw, Cheat (Cooper),
21

SATURN (Student Athlete Testing
Using Random Notification)
study, 77
Savulescu, Julian, 30–31
Selig, Bud, 68–69
Simpson, Tom, 13
Sosa, Sammy, 26
sports
drug testing ensures fairness in,
29–32
WADA on the spirit of, 14
stanozolol, 17
steroids. *See* anabolic steroids
Stinchcomb, Robert A., 7, 10, 35
surveys
of athletes, on drug testing, 53,
79
of colleges, on drugs tested for,
65
on drug testing as deterrent,
77–78
on drug use
among NCAA athletes, 74–75
by professional football/hockey
players, 29
of high schools
on drug testing, 57, 58
on penalties for drug use, 63

on treatment plans for athletes
testing positive, 66
of parents, on need for drug
testing, 60

Taylor Hooton Foundation, 37, 38
teens, performance-enhancing
drugs and, 35–37
testosterone, 9, 27, 34, 48
anabolic steroids and, 11
synthetic, 19
tetrahydrogestrinone (THG), 19,
68
Thorkildsen, Andreas, 27, 29–30
Tour de France, 6, 13, 15, 68,
72–73
drugs permitted by, 41–42
history of drug use in, 7–8
Trafton, Stephanie Brown, 47
Tygart, Travis, 46, 49

United States Anti-Doping Agency
(USADA), 6
University of Mainz, 79
University of Oregon, 55
University of Pennsylvania, 77

Verducci, Tom, 71
*Vernonia School District 47Jj v.
Acton* (1995), 54, 61
Volkow, Nora D., 36, 37

WADA. *See* World Anti-Doping
Agency (WADA)
weightlifting, 25
Wickerham, Andrea, 58
World Anti-Doping Agency
(WADA), 16, 17, 26, 53
on the spirit of sport, 14
substances banned by, 39–40, 43
World Anti-Doping Code, 14

Youth Risk Behavior Surveillance,
35

Picture Credits

About the Author

Lydia Bjornlund is a freelance writer and editor living in Northern Virginia. She has written more than two dozen nonfiction books for children and teens, mostly on American history and health-related topics. She also writes books and training materials for adults on issues related to land conservation, emergency management, and public policy. Bjornlund holds a master's degree in education from Harvard University and a BA in American Studies from Williams College. She lives with her husband, Gerry Hoetmer, and their children, Jake and Sophia.